CRYSTAL VISIONS

The Healing Power of Crystals

Roxayne Veasey

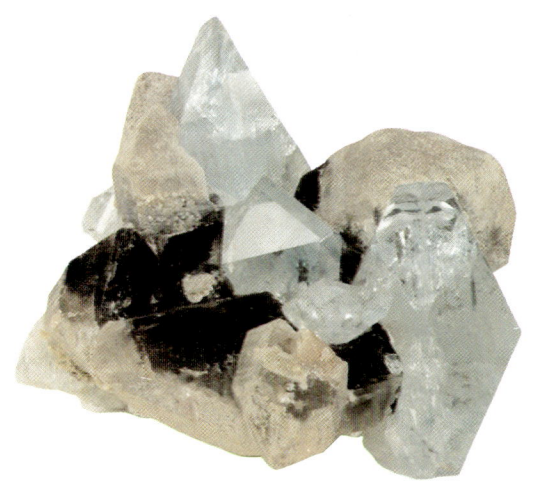

Whitford Press

77 Lower Valley Road
Atglen, Pennsylvania 19310 USA

DEDICATION

I dedicate this book to all the people who assisted me in it's creation.

Designed by Bonnie Hensley

Copyright © 1993 by Roxayne Veasey.
Library of Congress Catalog Number: 93-60017.

All rights reserved. No part of this work may be reproduced or used in any forms or by any means—graphic, electronic or mechanical, including photocopying or information storage and retrieval systems—without written permission from the copyright holder.

Printed in the United States of America.
ISBN: 0-924608-15-3

We are interested in hearing from authors with book ideas on related topics.

Published by Whitford Press

A Division of Schiffer Publishing, Ltd.
77 Lower Valley Road
Atglen, PA 19310
Please write for a free catalog.
This book may be purchased from the publisher.
Please include $2.95 postage.

ACKNOWLEDGEMENTS

Sarah and Christopher Culley for being my inspiration.
Dottie and Bill Veasey for always being interested.
Alena Heble, for support in creating and typing manuscript.
Peter Redmond, for his willingnes in teaching and healing me.
Dave Johnson, thank you for your advice.
Isis Crisis Jewelry, use of crystals and stones.
Dr. Peter Levine access to the collection of Dupont minerals at the University of Del.,
for many of the photographs in this book.
Rosemary Lane, use of crystals.
Larry Zaleski, D.C., use of crystals.
Mark Weisberg, use of crystals.
Jeffrey B. Snyder, thank you for exquisite photography and editing.
All my family I love you for your support.
The Devas of the Mineral Kingdom for sharing their light with the world.

INTRODUCTION

CRYSTAL VISIONS has been designed to identify minerals, reveal some general information about their makeup and occurrence, and give a basic appreciation and application of their specific healing properties. I believe the basis of disease is in the disharmony caused by conflicting moods within the spiritual and mental aspects of a human being. These moods lower the body's innate vitality and allow for dis-ease to be present.

When a mineral is placed on or around the body the vibration of the body is affected. This phenomenon is called attuning to the crystal vibration.

In this book the crystals and stones are associated with specific body zones called chakras. There are seven major chakras on the body which correspond with seven major glands in the endocrine system.

In order to do a full body attunement you will choose seven crystals or stones with the appropriate color and healing properties you want to add to your body's vibration and place them on your chakras for half an hour. During the attunement you should be relaxed and quiet. Enjoy the strength of the crystals and stones as they share their vibrations with you.

CONTENTS

Acknowledgements 3

Introduction 4

Chapter One 7

   AGATE—BLUE LACE, BOTSWANA, MOSS 7

   AMBER 10

   AMETHYST 11

   AQUAMARINE 13

   AVENTURINE 15

   AZURITE 16

   BLOODSTONE 18

   CALCITE—WHITE, HONEY, GREEN, PINK, PEACH 19

   CARNELIAN 22

   CELESTITE 24

   CHRYSOCOLLA 26

   CITRINE 27

   DIAMOND—CLEAR, BLUE, YELLOW 28

   EMERALD 30

   FLOURITE—BLUE, GREEN, PURPLE 32

   GARNET 34

   HAWK'S EYE 35

   HEMATITE 36

JADITE	37
KAYANITE	39
KUNZITE	40
LAPIS LAZULI	42
MALACHITE	44
MOLDAVITE	46
MOONSTONE	47
OBSIDIAN—GOLDEN SHEEN, BLACK, SNOWFLAKE	48
PERIDOT	50
PYRITE	51
QUARTZ—ROSE, RUTILATED, SKELETAL, SMOKEY, TOURMALATED	53
RHODOCHROSITE	59
RUBY	61
SAPPHIRE	62
SELENITE	63
SODOLITE	66
SULFUR	67
TIGER'S EYE	68
TOPAZ	69
TOURMALINE—BLACK, BLUE, PINK, GREEN, WATERMELON	71
TURQUOISE	76
Chapter Two	77
Cross References	77

CHAPTER ONE

AGATE

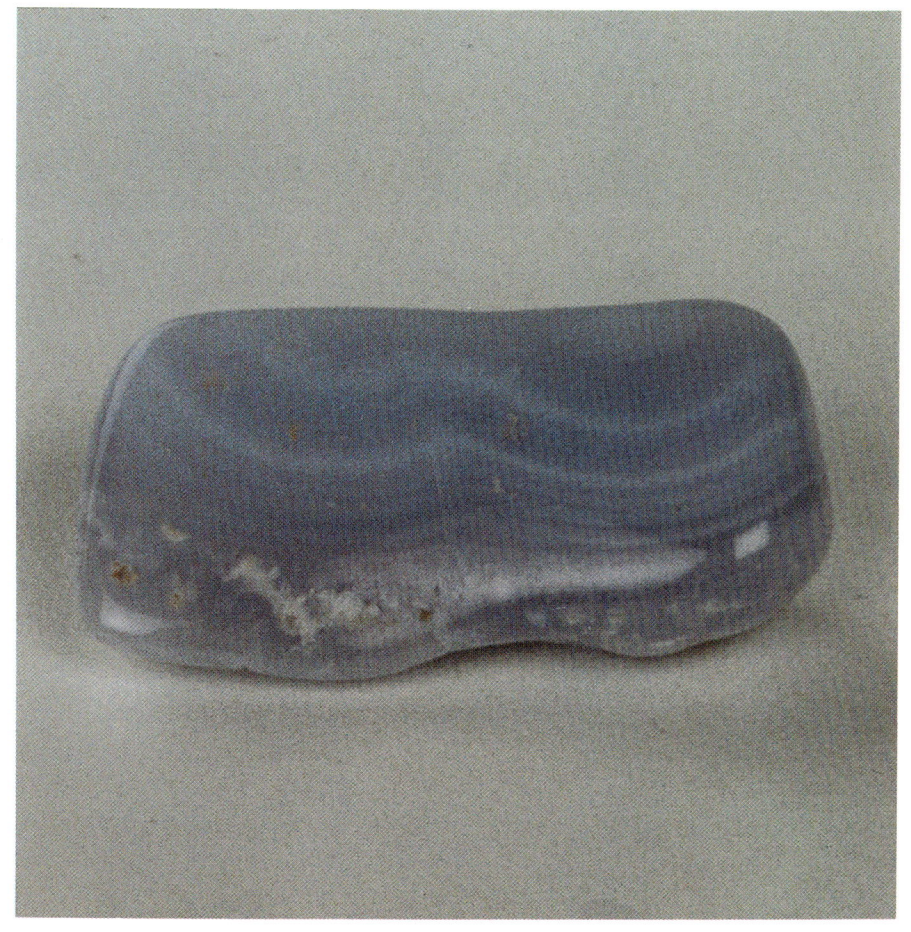

BLUE LACE AGATE

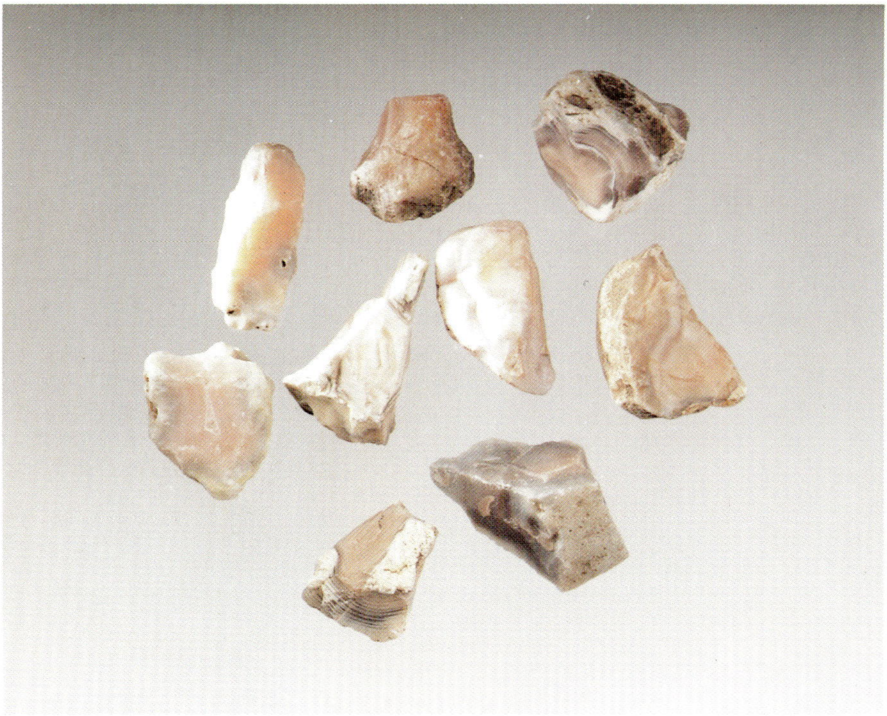

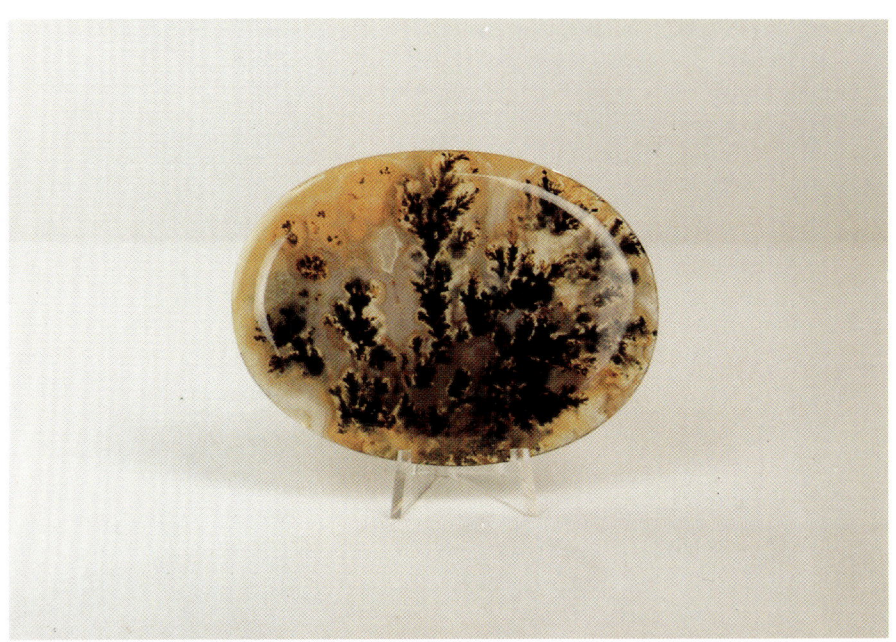

BOTSWANA AGATE

MOSS AGATE

Agate is a microcrystalline variety of quartz with consecutive layers of many colors. Germany and Italy are more famous for agates than any other country.

Agates are some of the most beautiful stones. They have an earthy quality, I often carry agates to experience my connection with Mother Earth.

HEALING PROPERTIES

BLUE LACE AGATE

AIDS THE FLOW OF SELF EXPRESSION
ASSISTS IN LOVING COMMUNICATION
RELIEVES NECK AND SHOULDER PAIN
ALLEVIATES HEADACHES
HEALS SORE THROATS
AIDS THYROID PROBLEMS
NEUTRALIZES ANGER, INFLAMMATION AND INFECTIONS

SIXTH CHAKRA STONE

BOTSWANA AGATE

AMPLIFIES THE
COLOR AND VIBRATION OF OTHER STONES

ALL CHAKRA STONE

MOSS AGATE

IMPROVES BLOOD
CIRCULATION
AIDS CIRCULATION OF THE LYMPH SYSTEM
LENDS HARMONY IN THE ENVIRONMENT

ALL CHAKRA STONE

AMBER

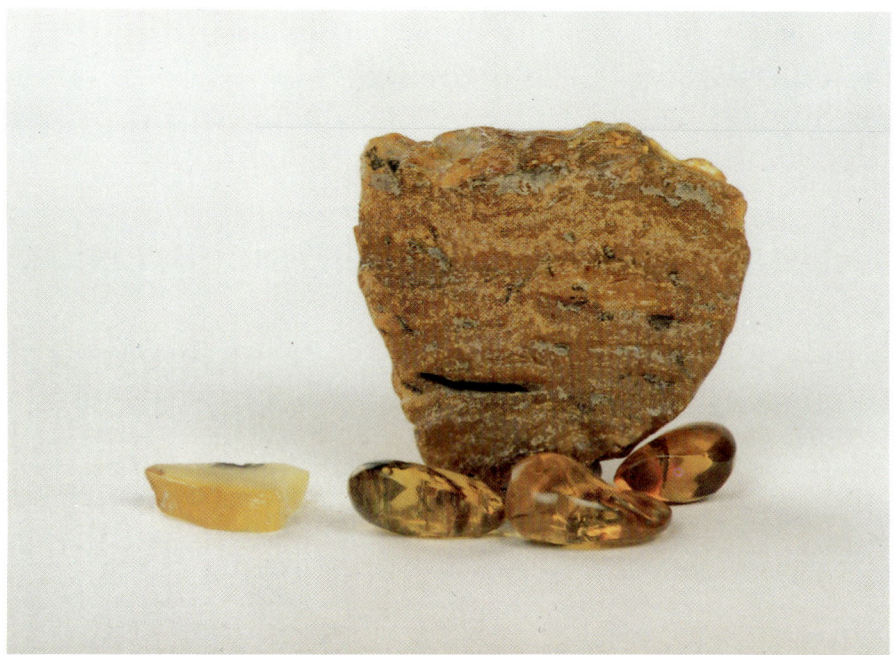

Amber is soft and very light, often containing pieces of fossilized remains of plants and insects. It is transparent and ranges in color from a golden yellow, to a deep red, and a dark brown. Romania, Italy, Spain, the former Soviet Union, Canada, and Poland are the primary sources of amber.

I am wildly attracted to amber with it's warm and sensuous color. Although amber is not a crystal or stone, it's healing properties have been reported since the beginning of time.

HEALING PROPERTIES

**STRENGTHENS TISSUES OF THE CENTRAL NERVOUS SYSTEM
DRAINS DISEASE OUT OF THE TISSUES OF THE BODY
ABSORBS NEGATIVE ENERGY, STIMULATES ALL THE GLANDS IN THE BODY**

ALL CHAKRA STONE

AMETHYST

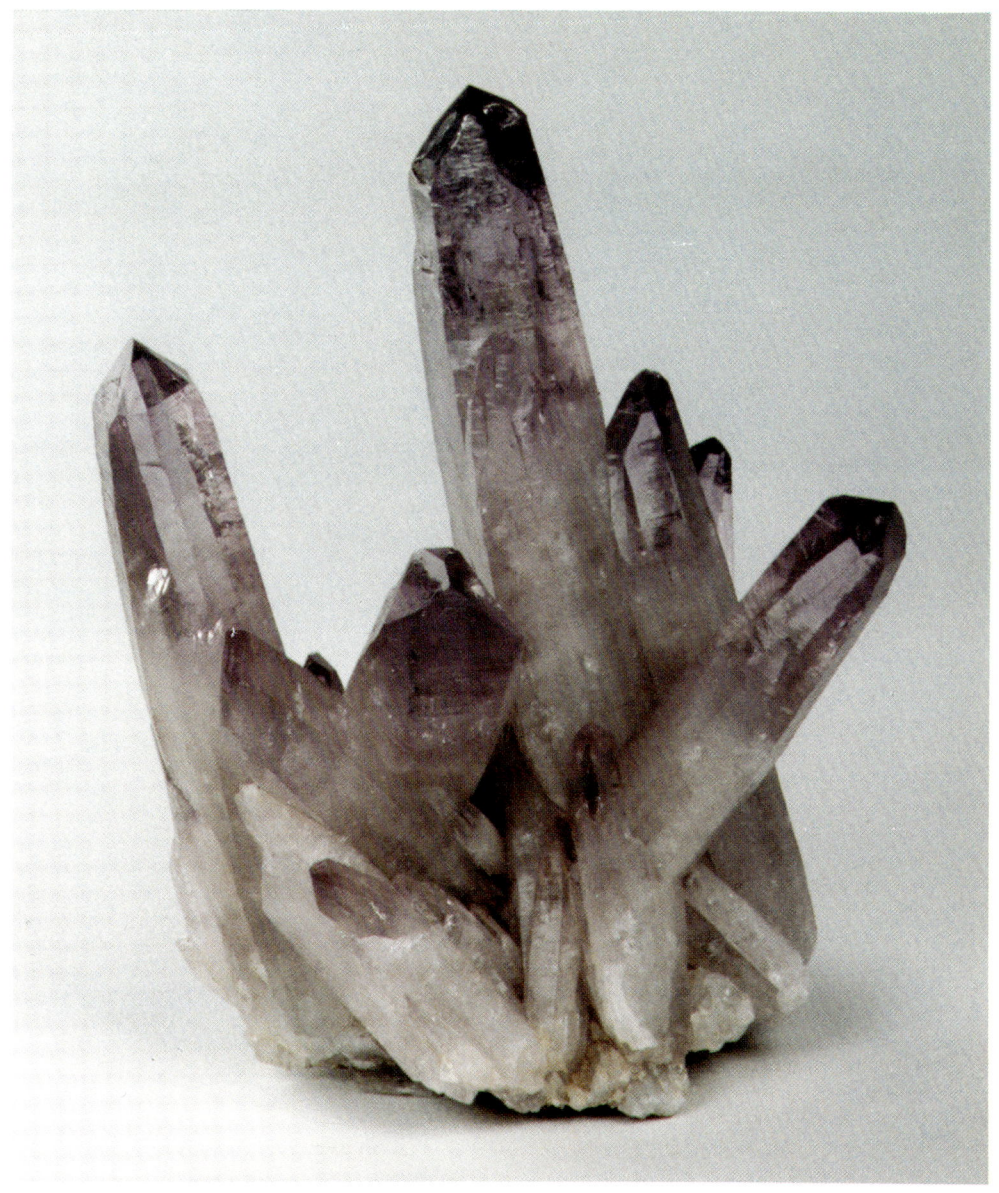

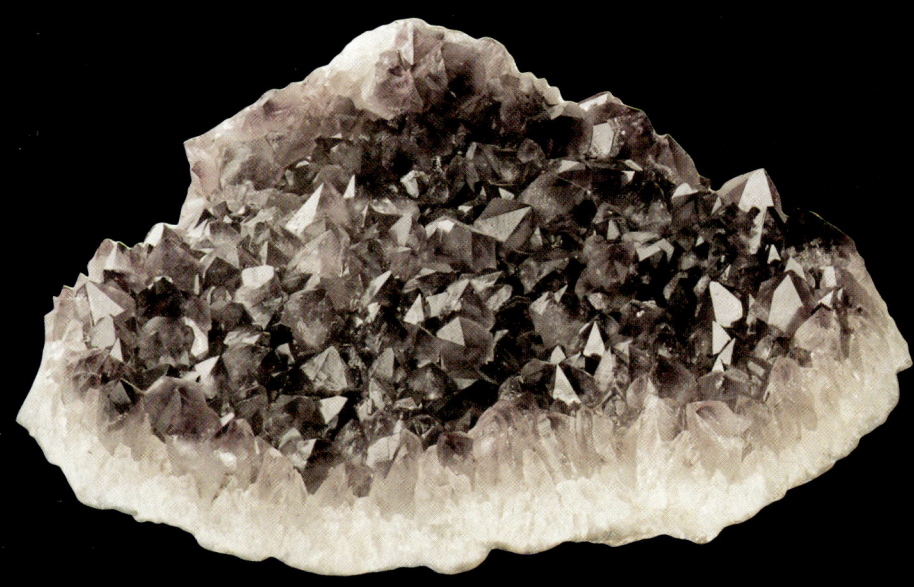

Amethyst is part of the quartz family, whose color varies from a pale violet to a dark, rich purple. Although amethyst is mined in many countries, the finest crystals are found in Brazil and Uruguay. This is the most highly prized variety of quartz.

The family room is a good place to have a large cluster of amethyst to disperse any negative vibrations that may accumulate.

HEALING PROPERTIES

CALMS THE MIND FOR MEDITATION OR SLEEP
REPELS NEGATIVITY AND LENDS PROTECTION
RELEASES OLD EMOTIONAL THOUGHT PATTERNS
STIMULATES PINEAL AND PITUITARY GLANDS

SIXTH AND SEVENTH CHAKRA CRYSTAL

AQUAMARINE

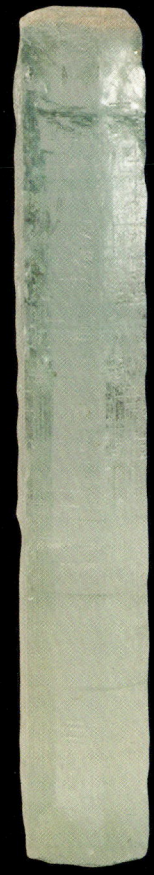

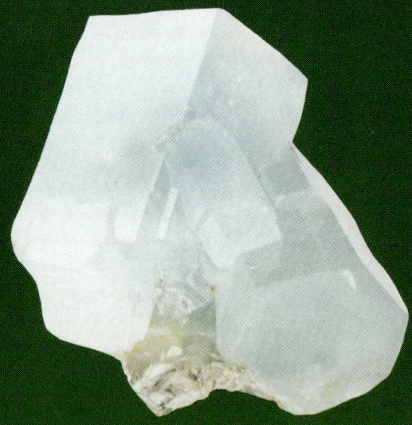

Aquamarine is a gem stone whose watery blue-green color is due to the iron content. The sky blue color is the most valuable even though the blue has a tinge of green. The most famous aquamarine comes from Brazil, with other deposits occurring in Madagascar, the former Soviet Union, the United States, and Afghanistan.

Among the healing properties of aquamarine are releasing both fear and fluid. I found this interesting because I had suspected fluid retention was associated with the letting go of fears.

HEALING PROPERTIES

USEFUL IN REDUCING FLUID RETENTION
ACTIVATES THE THYMUS GLAND
AIDS IN CREATIVE EXPRESSION
PRODUCES CLARITY OF THOUGHT PROCESS
DISSIPATES FEARS AND PHOBIAS

THIRD AND FIFTH CHAKRA CRYSTAL

AVENTURINE

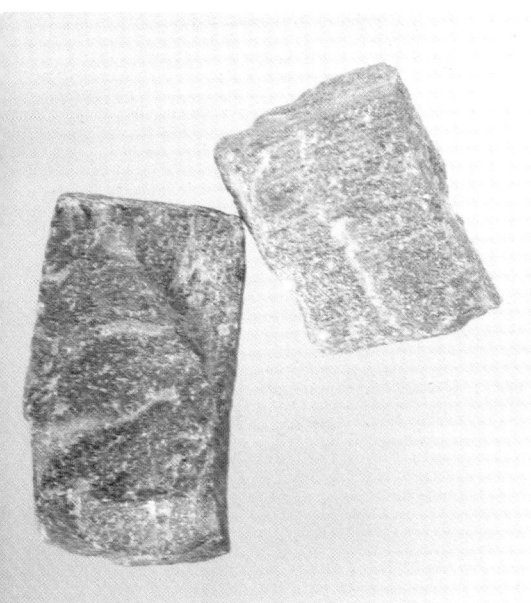 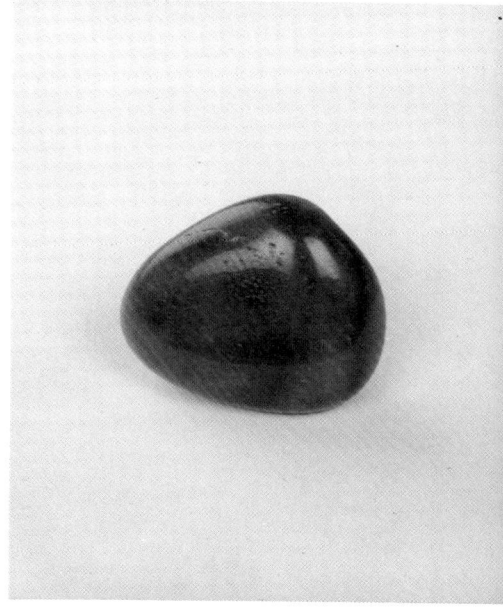

Aventurine is in the quartz family. It has a granular appearance and ranges in color from a brownish-yellow to green. It is found in the United States, Mexico, Germany and Japan.

Children are very attracted to this stone. I often suggest that they carry a tumbled piece in their pockets and rub it for comfort.

HEALING PROPERTIES

RELEASES EMOTIONAL STRESS
RELIEVES ANXIETY
STIMULATES MUSCLE TISSUE
STRENGTHENS THE BLOOD
RADIATES A POSITIVE ATTITUDE INTO THE ENVIRONMENT

FOURTH CHAKRA STONE

AZURITE

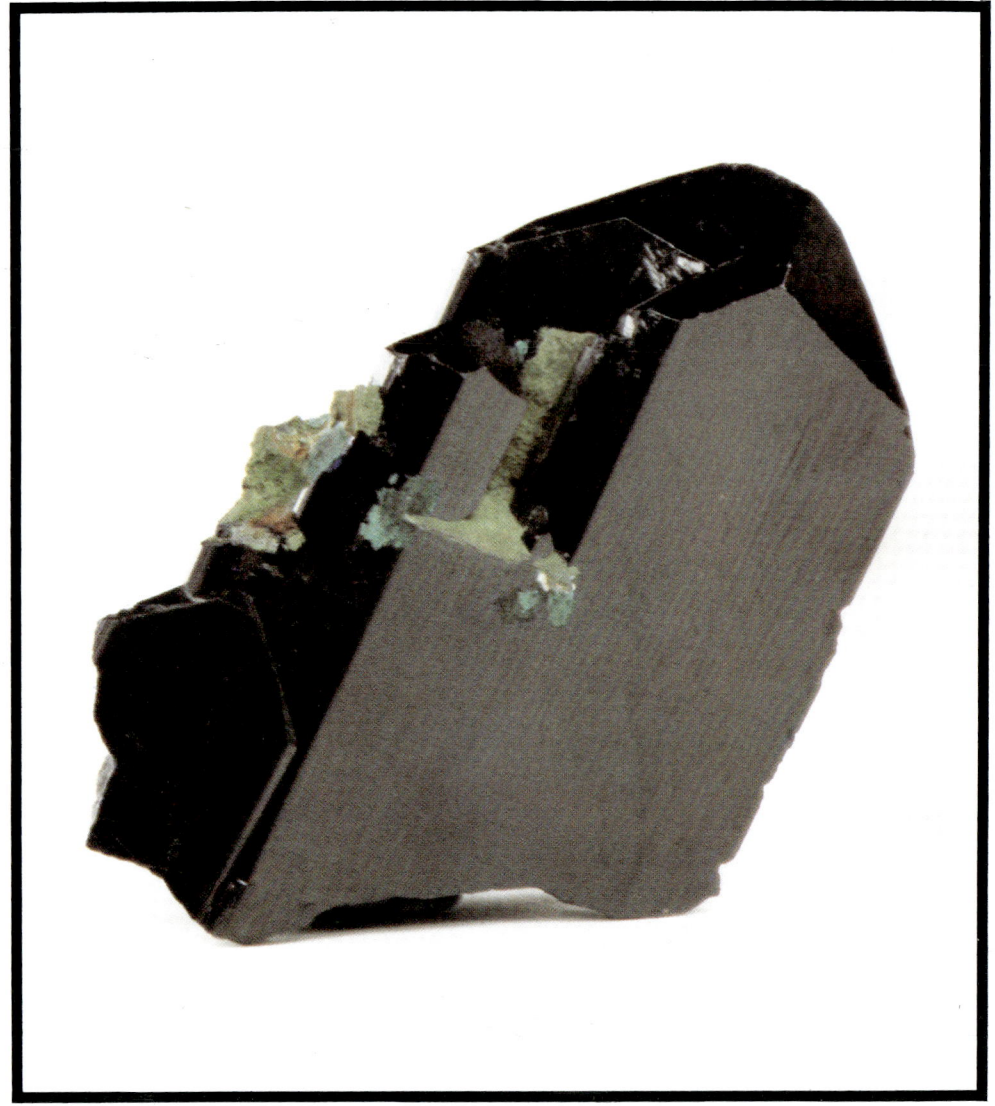

Azurite is a semi—hard, striated, elongated, or tabular prismatic crystal. The finest crystals are found in the United States, Greece, and France. This crystal is dark blue in color ranging to green as it becomes malachite.

This is the most exquisite crystal in the world for color and brilliance. Spend time meditating with this crystal on the sixth chakra and you will find it easier to read peoples' thoughts.

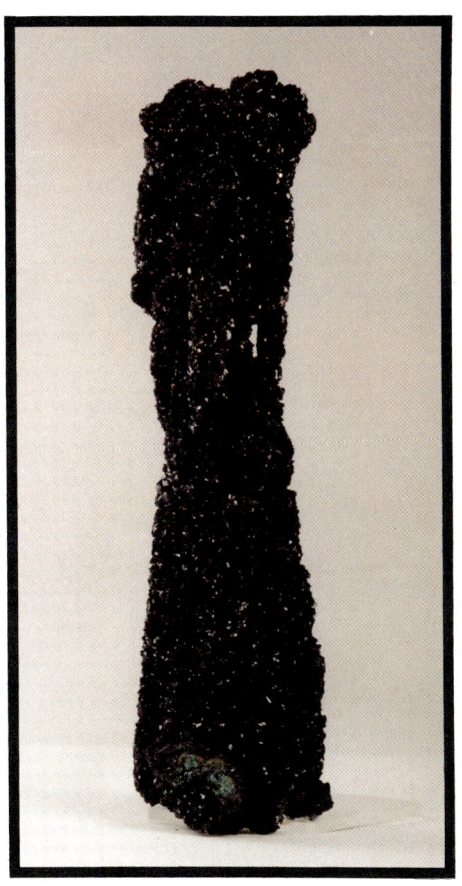

HEALING PROPERTIES

**STIMULATES PSYCHIC ABILITIES
IMPROVES VISUALIZATION
STIMULATES THE THYROID GLANDS
STIMULATING TO THE SPLEEN
CLEARS OLD THOUGHT PATTERNS**

FIFTH AND SIXTH CHAKRA CRYSTAL

BLOODSTONE

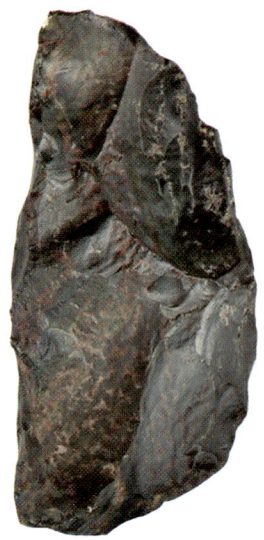

Bloodstone is a form of jasper with prominent reddish flecks throughout the primarily green stone. It is found in the United States and England where it is formed with volcanic solutions and ocean water.

In my house if something hurts, first we try a hug and if it still hurts we use the bloodstone. After you use the bloodstone you should always soak it.

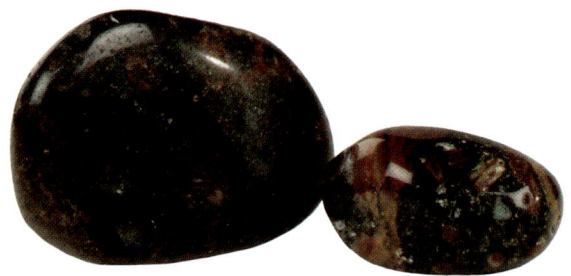

HEALING PROPERTIES

**GROUNDING
CLEANSES THE PHYSICAL BODY
HEALING FOR ALL BLOOD DISORDERS
RADIATES COURAGE INTO THE ENVIRONMENT
STRENGTHENS THE HEART, SPLEEN, AND BONE MARROW
STIMULATES THE FLOW OF KUNDALINI**

FIRST CHAKRA STONE

CALCITE

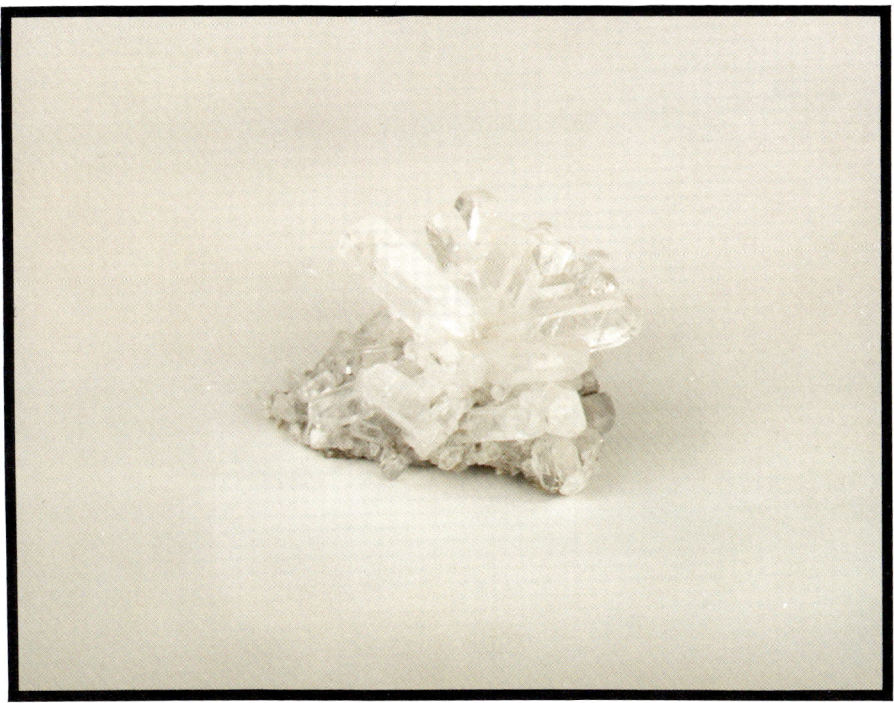

WHITE/TRANSPARENT CALCITE

HEALING PROPERTIES

**IMPROVES MEMORY
AIDS IN ASTRAL TRAVEL
HEALING FOR THE EYESIGHT
HELPS TO OBSERVE CLEARLY OR IN A NEW WAY**

SEVENTH CHAKRA CRYSTAL

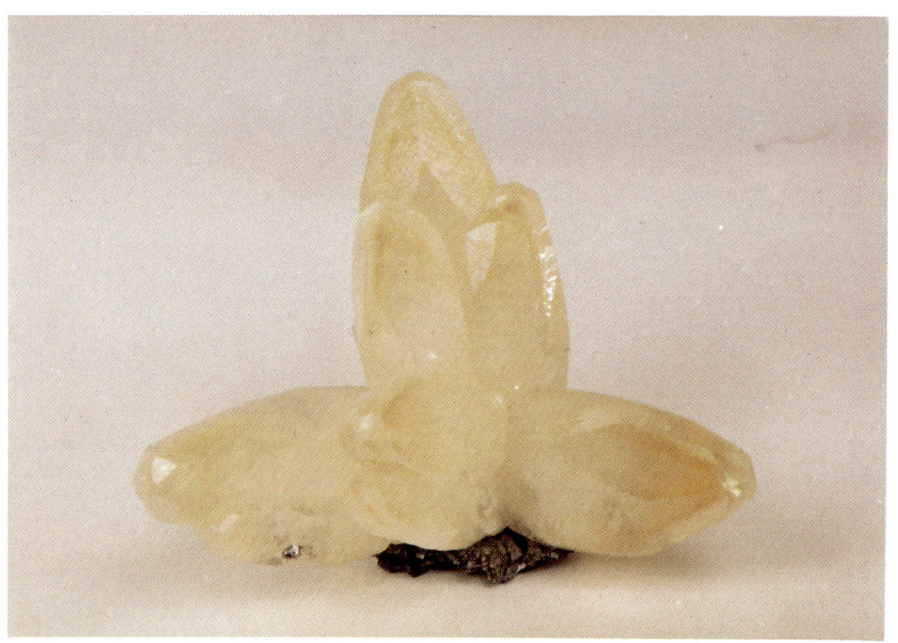

HONEY CALCITE

HEALING PROPERTIES

**STIMULATES THE KIDNEYS AND ELIMINATES BODY TOXINS
HELPS TO PROJECT CREATIVE THOUGHT INTO PHYSICAL REALITY
HEALING FOR THE GALL BLADDER
CALMS THE DIGESTIVE SYSTEM**

THIRD AND SEVENTH CHAKRA CRYSTAL

GREEN CALCITE

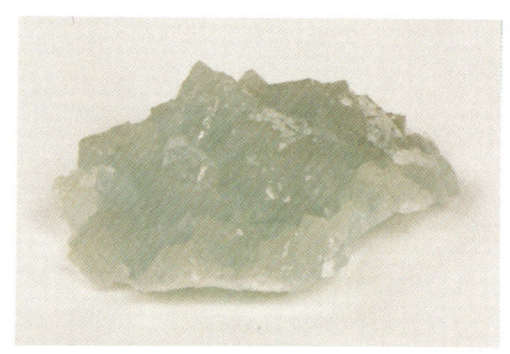

HEALING PROPERTIES

**MENTAL HEALING
HELPS RELEASE RIGID MENTAL PATTERNS AND ALLOWS FOR NEW POSSIBILITIES**

SIXTH CHAKRA CRYSTAL

PEACH CALCITE

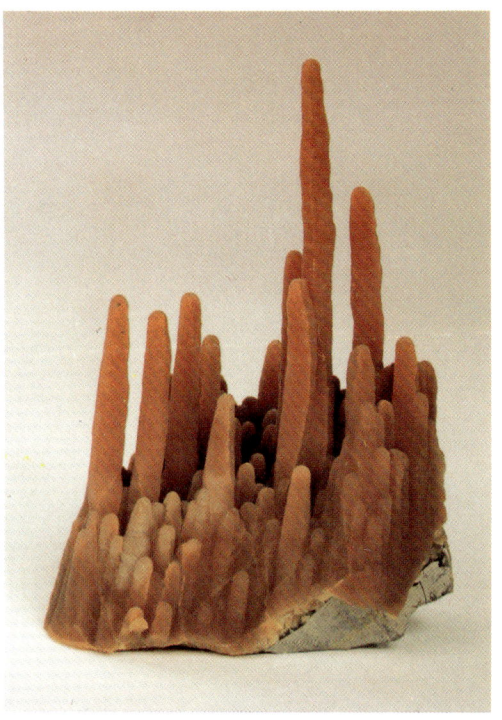

HEALING PROPERTIES

**EXPANDS THE CAPACITY OF LOVE
DISSOLVES SADNESS AND GRIEF
LENDS UNCONDITIONAL LOVE WHEN PLACED IN THE ENVIRONMENT**

ALL CHAKRA CRYSTAL

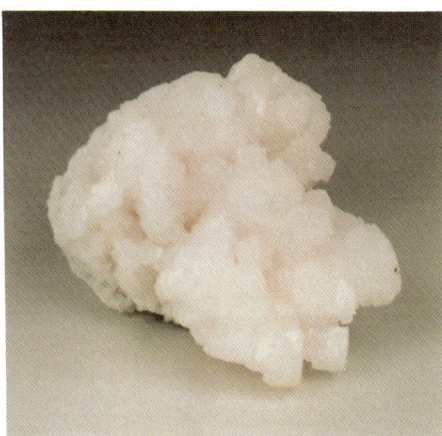

PINK CALCITE

HEALING PROPERTIES

**BLENDS THE ENERGIES OF THE HEART AND THE MIND
USEFUL CRYSTAL FOR MEDITATION
OPENS CHAKRAS THIRD THROUGH SEVENTH
HEALS WILLPOWER ISSUES**

THIRD, FIFTH, AND SEVENTH CHAKRA CRYSTAL

Calcite color occurs as transparent, white, pink, red, green, yellow, and blue. The forms of calcite are varied, ranging from prismatic, scalenohedral, rhombohedral, and in masses often intergrown. It is found in Iceland, Italy, Germany, the United States, England, Hungary, Mexico, and the former Soviet Union.

Calcite of any type really helps out at homework time. Because this is a crystal of the heart and mind it is also useful by the telephone.

CARNELIAN

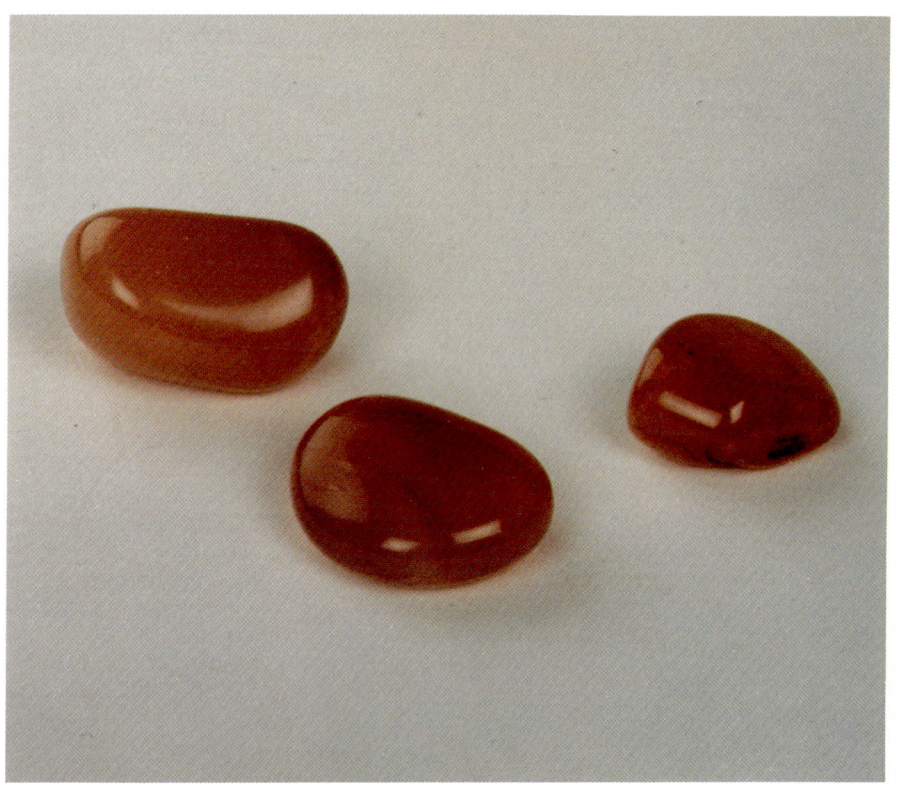

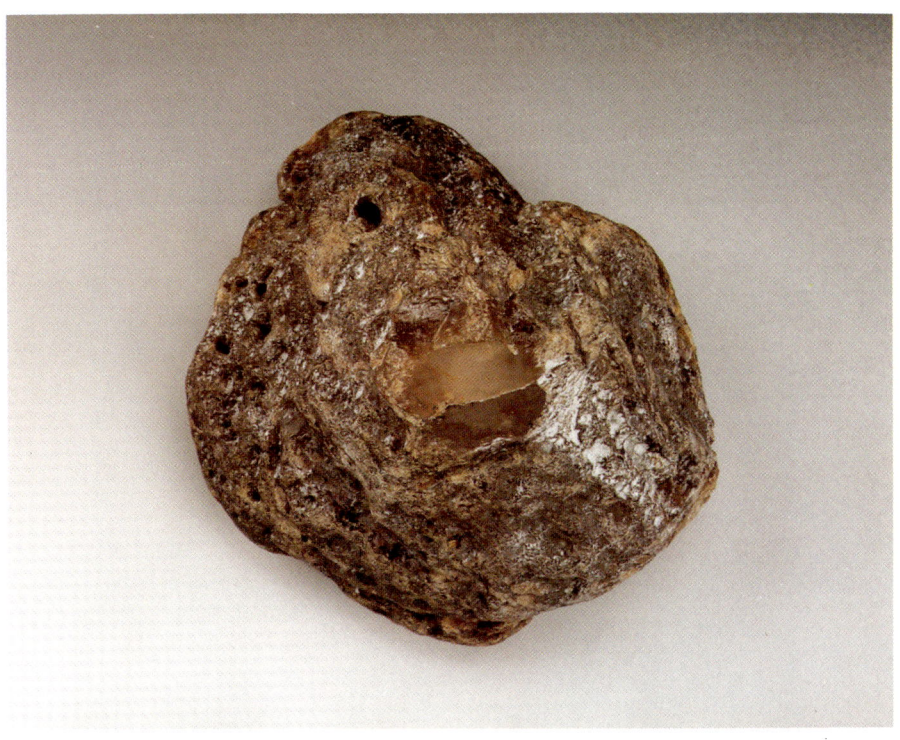

Carnelian is a microcrystalline variety of quartz that forms in concretionary deposits. Large amounts come from Uruguay, and Brazil although it is found in many other countries.

If you have a child or friend that is unsure of themselves, carnelian would make a wonderful gift. A piece of jewelry or a tumbled pocket stone to carry should do the trick.

HEALING PROPERTIES

**HELPS ACTUALIZE PERSONAL POWER IN THE PHYSICAL PLANE
ASSISTS IN RELIEF FOR ASTHMATIC SYMPTOMS**

SECOND CHAKRA CRYSTAL

CELESTITE

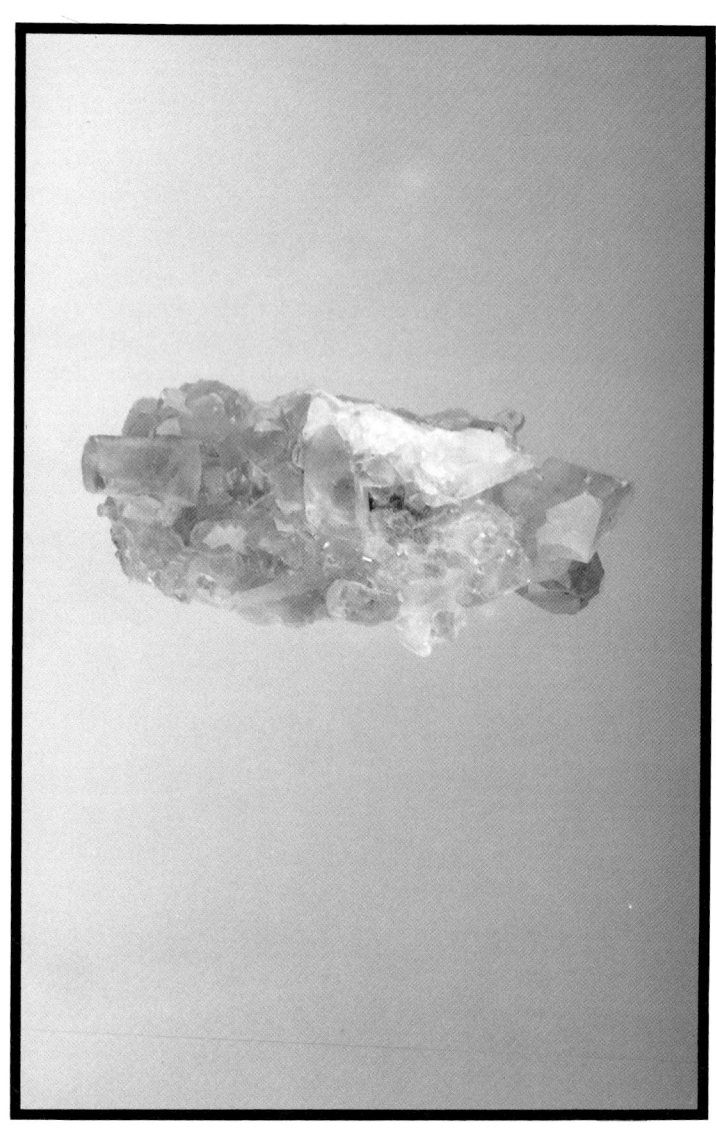

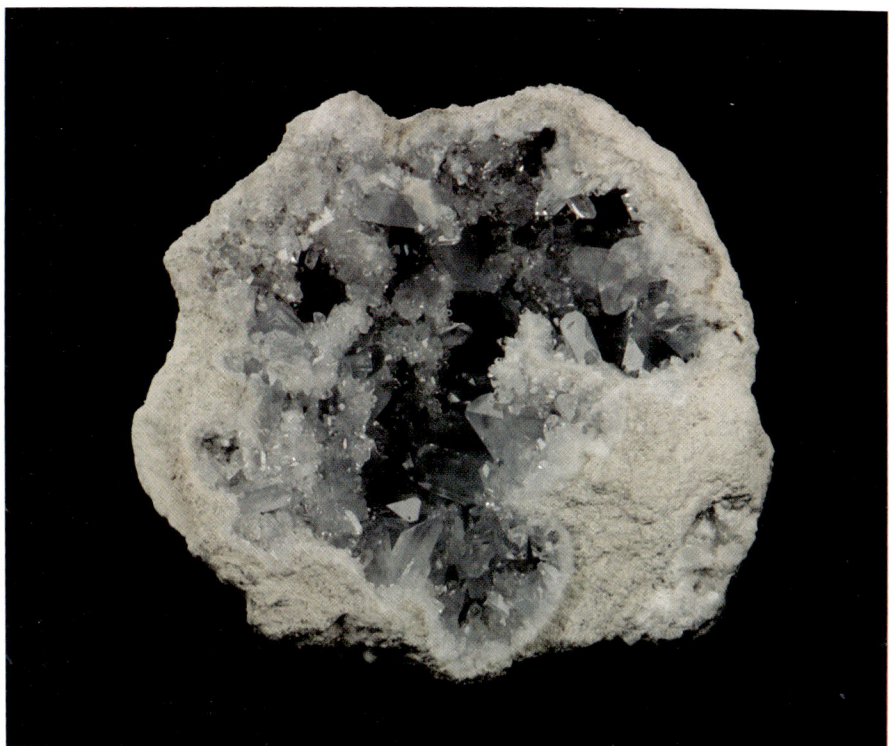

Celestite commonly forms as prismatic and occasionally as tabular crystals. The transparent to translucent colors are clear, white, pale blue, and yellow. It is found in Italy, England, the United States, and the former Soviet Union.

Celestite, as its name suggests, has a celestial vibration. It is useful in meditation, particularly if you wish to contact the angelic realms.

HEALING PROPERTIES

RELIEVES TENSION HEADACHES
IMPROVES COMMUNICATION SKILLS
ENHANCES THYROID FUNCTION
AIDS PERSONAL CREATIVITY
RAISES CONSCIOUSNESS

FIFTH CHAKRA CRYSTAL

CHRYSOCOLLA

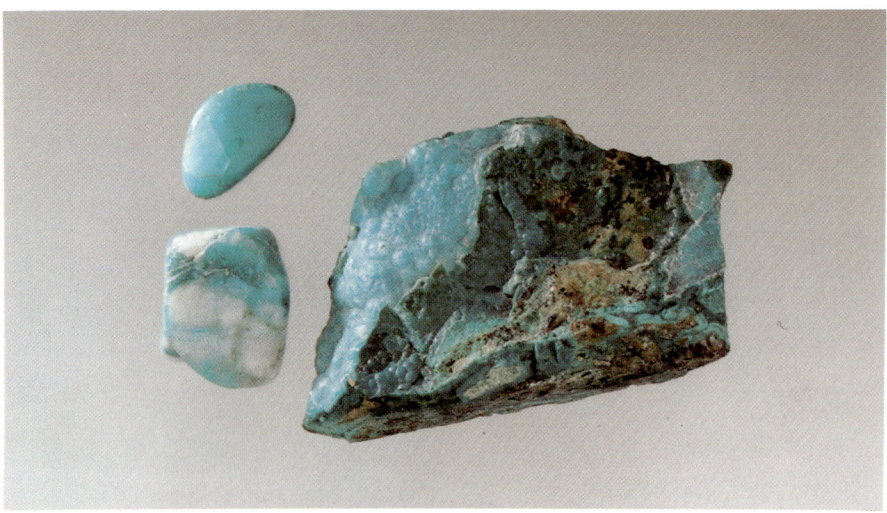

Chrysocolla is formed in stalactite masses or in microcrystalline slabs. It is a soft stone that is a bright green to blue and is often found near copper deposits. It is found in Chile, the United States, Morocco, Rhodesia, the former Soviet Union, and Italy.

This is a stone with distinct feminine energies that is sometimes referred to as gem silica. Meditating or bathing with gem silica can put you in touch with your own feminine nature.

HEALING PROPERTIES

RELEASES STRESS
STRENGTHENS LUNGS
STIMULATES THYROID GLAND
REDUCES ANGER, FEAR AND GUILT
AID FOR FEMALE DISORDERS
HELPS CLEAR SUBCONSCIOUS IMBALANCES
BALANCES UPPER AND LOWER CHAKRAS

FOURTH AND FIFTH CHAKRA CRYSTAL

CITRINE

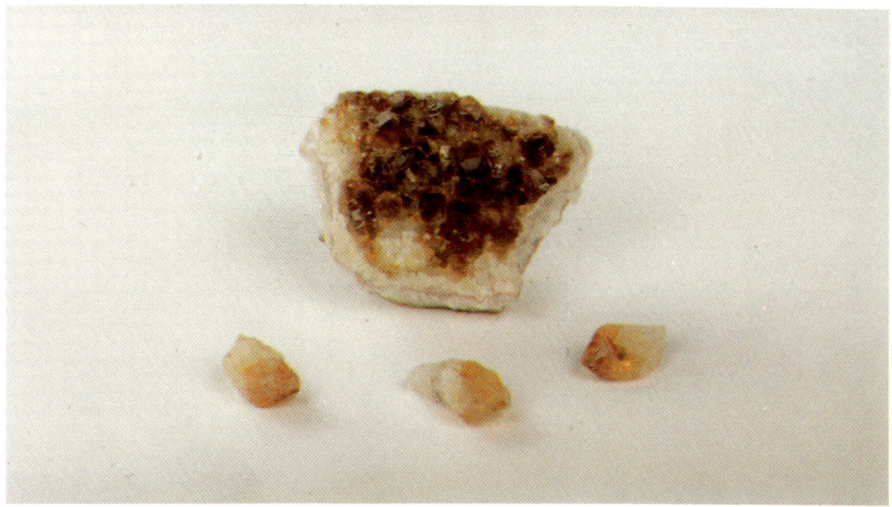

The color of citrine is yellow or brown depending on the inclusions of iron hydrates. It is a member of the quartz family found in Brazil, France, and the former Soviet Union.

Citrine would be a valuable gift to someone who has problems with addictive behavior. It helps to restore personal power and lends needed healing.

HEALING PROPERTIES

ENHANCES THE BODY'S INNATE HEALING ENERGY
DETOXIFIES THE BODY
REGENERATES BODY TISSUES
REDUCES SELF-DESTRUCTIVE TENDENCIES
INCREASES INTUITION

THIRD AND SEVENTH CHAKRA CRYSTAL

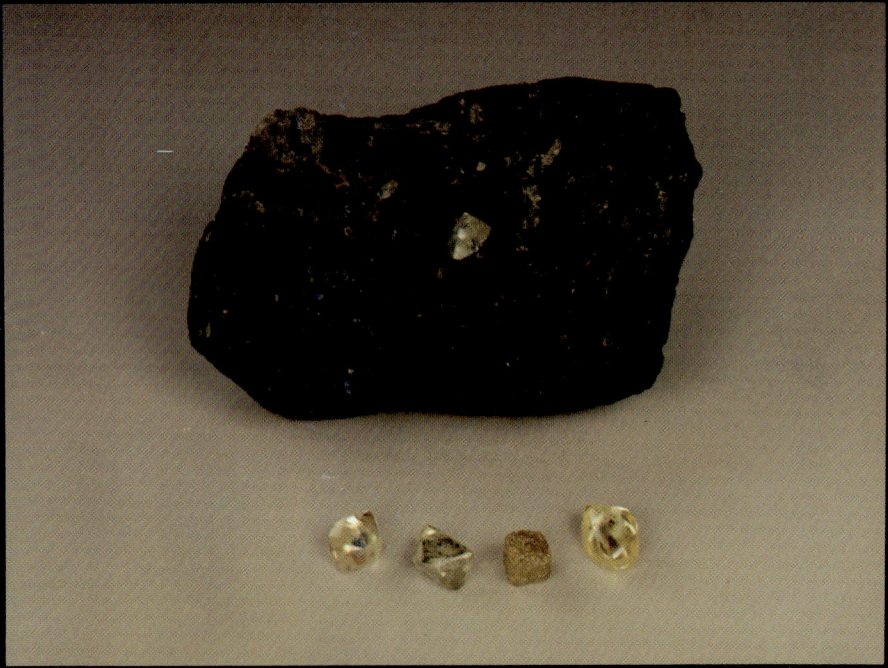

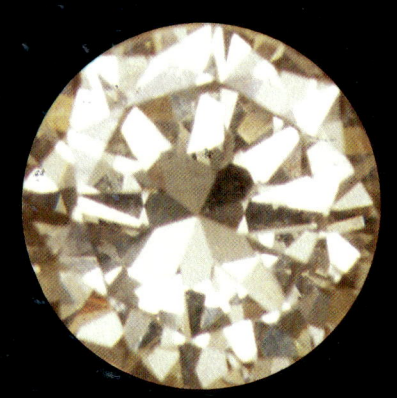

The color of diamonds run the entire spectrum from perfectly clear, to pink, yellow, blue, green, and violet. Mined only in India for centuries, diamond crystals are found in Brazil, South Africa, the former Soviet Union, Venezuela, and China.

The diamond vibration is about the outward expression of personal power. If you have a presentation or important meeting to attend, wear your diamonds.

HEALING PROPERTIES

CLEAR DIAMOND
**CLEARS SEVENTH CHAKRA
ENHANCES BRAIN FUNCTION
DISPELS NEGATIVITY
ADDS ALIGNMENT WITH HIGHER SELF**

ALL CHAKRA CRYSTAL

YELLOW DIAMOND

**CHARGES PERSONAL POWER
EXPANDS CONSCIOUSNESS**

THIRD AND SEVENTH CHAKRA CRYSTAL

BLUE DIAMOND
**BRILLIANT COMMUNICATION
RELEASES WITHHELD COMMUNICATION**

FIFTH CHAKRA CRYSTAL

EMERALD

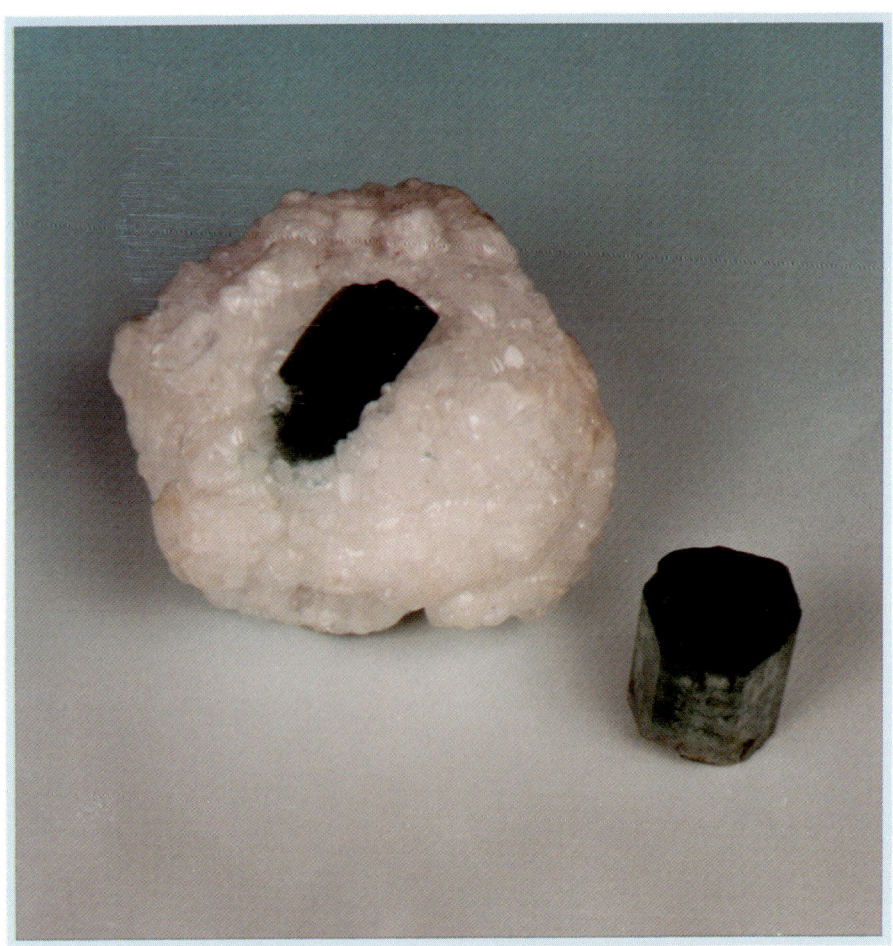

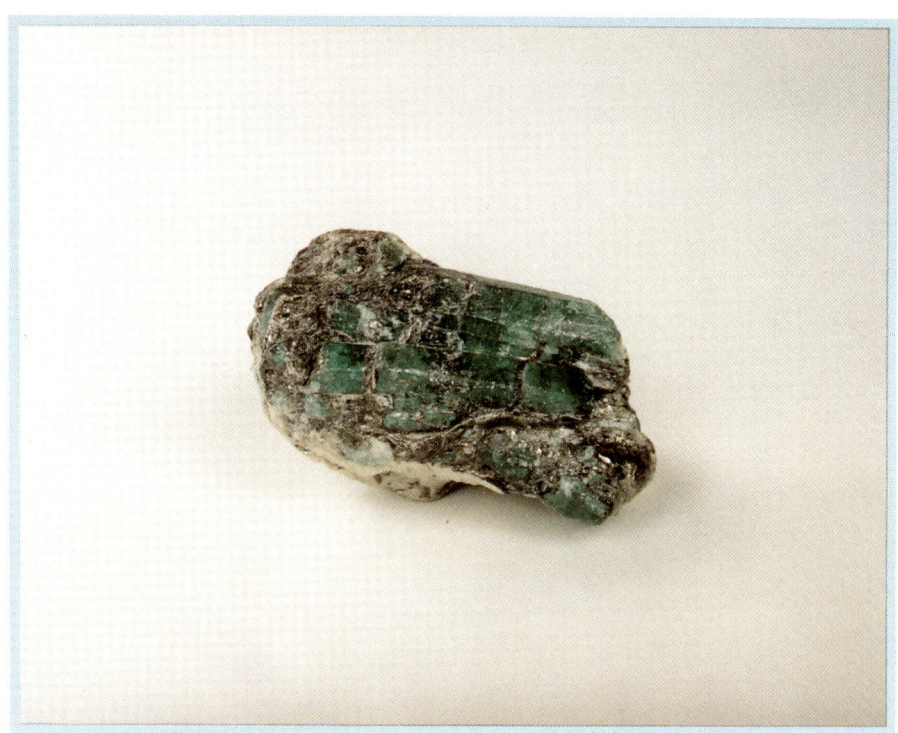

Emeralds can be light to dark green. The color is due to chromium in the crystal structure. The mines in Columbia produce the world's most beautiful emeralds. Brazil, Africa, India, and Pakistan extract emeralds of lesser quality.

The color most often associated with healing is emerald green. Just visualizing this color can have a powerful affect on the body and mind continuum.

HEALING PROPERTIES

CALMING EFFECT ON THE MIND
REDUCES EYESTRAIN
STRENGTHENS IMMUNE AND NERVOUS SYSTEMS
STRONG BALANCE FOR EMOTIONS

FOURTH CHAKRA CRYSTAL

FLORITE

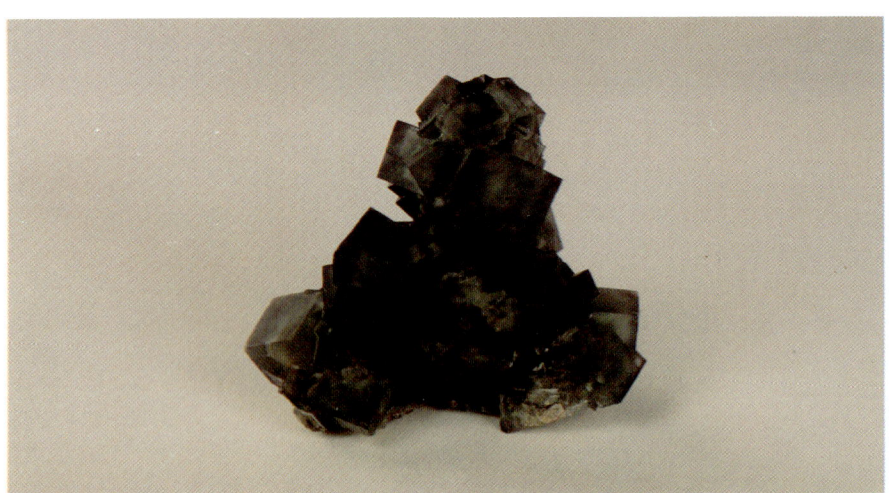

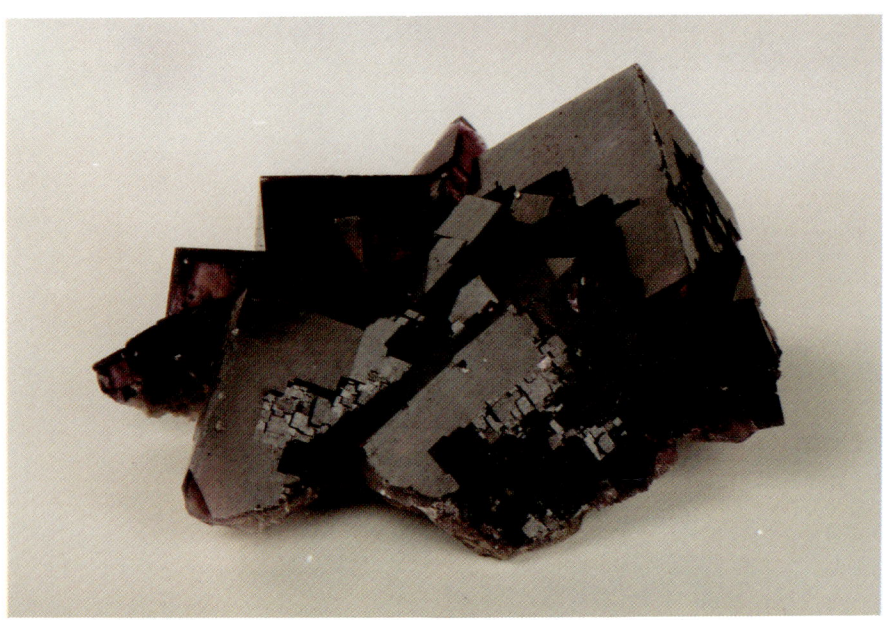

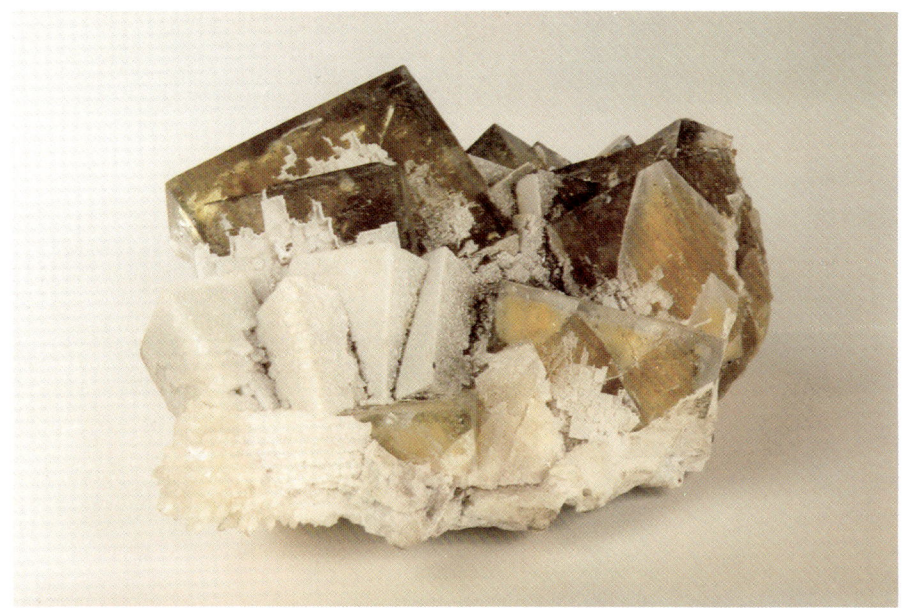

Florite forms in cubes, octohedrals and dodecahedrals, and may be found in masses that are compacted or banded. The color is extremely variable. Florite is transparent, yellow, green, blue, pink, purple, or even black. It can be found in Italy, Switzerland, the United States, Norway, Canada, Germany, and England.

Every office should come equipped with florite to relieve mental stress. If you or someone you love works in an office, a florite paperweight is a must.

BLUE/GREEN/PURPLE FLORITE

HEALING PROPERTIES

**FACILITATES INTERDIMENSIONAL COMMUNICATION
BALANCES MENTAL ENERGIES
AIDS MEDITATIVE STATE OF MIND
RELIEVES MENTAL STRESS
AIDS UNDERSTANDING OF ABSTRACT CONCEPTS
HEALING FOR STROKES AND ARTHRITIS
GROUNDS ENERGY/HYPER-ACTIVITY**

SIXTH AND SEVENTH CHAKRA CRYSTAL

GARNET

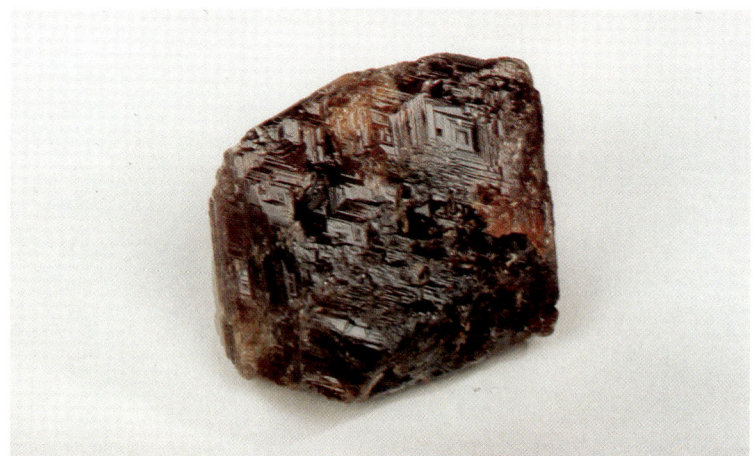

Garnet is a deep red that tends toward brown, it can also be a deep violet-red. Garnets are found mainly in Sri Lanka and India with other sources in Burma, the United States, Madagascar, Brazil, and Austria.

Although garnets occur in a variety of colors, red is the one most often used for the purposes of attuning to the crystal vibrations. Garnets' rich red color lends the property of grounding to scattered energies.

HEALING PROPERTIES

RED GARNET
STIMULATES BLOOD FLOW
AIDS IN HEALING ANEMIA
HARMONIZES THE FLOW OF KUNDALINI
STIMULATES THE PITUITARY GLAND
GROUNDING

FIRST CHAKRA CRYSTAL

HAWK'S EYE

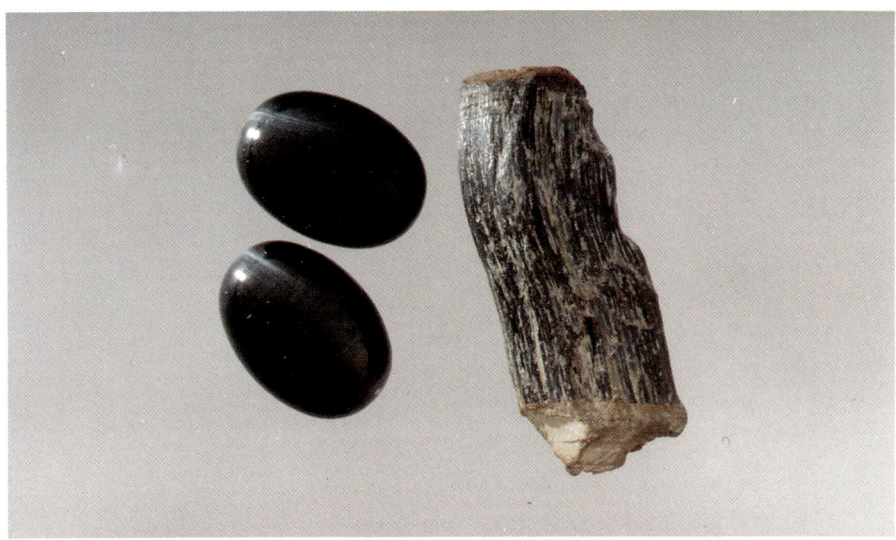

Hawk's eye is a blue or blue-grey fibrous inclusion in a quartz base with a mobile reflection. It is found mainly in South Africa.

If you would like to feel more secure about your episodes of extrasensory perceptions, this stone can be an invaluable aid.

HEALING PROPERTIES

"SEER STONE"
HELPFUL IN GAINING THE PROPER PERSPECTIVE
LENDS PEACE IN ITS ENVIRONMENT
PLEASANTLY GROUNDING

FIRST CHAKRA CRYSTAL

HEMATITE

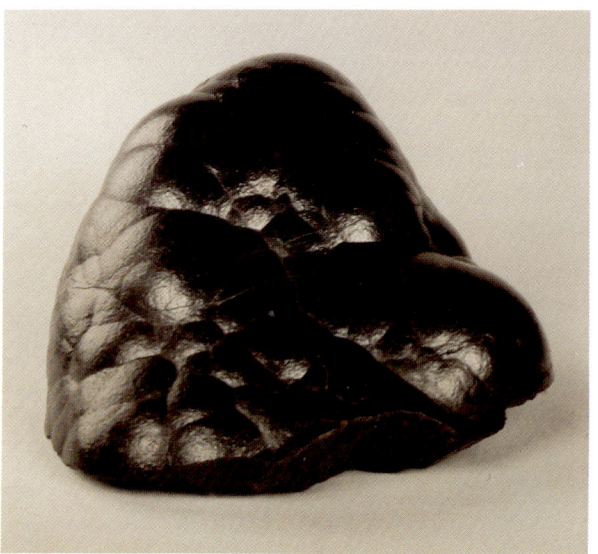 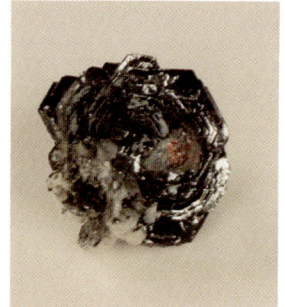

While hematite occasionally occurs as black rombohedral crystals, it is more often found in compact masses with iridescent coloring on the surface. This stone is found in the United States, Canada, Venezuela, Brazil, Angola, the former Soviet Union, England, and Switzerland.

When a client complains of feeling "spaced-out" I recommend they carry a few tumbled stones of hematite. This will help them to feel grounded and reduce their stress level.

HEALING PROPERTIES

ACTIVATES SPLEEN
INCREASES RESISTANCE TO STRESS
GROUNDING
TRANSFORMS NEGATIVE ENERGY TO POSITIVE

FIRST CHAKRA CRYSTAL

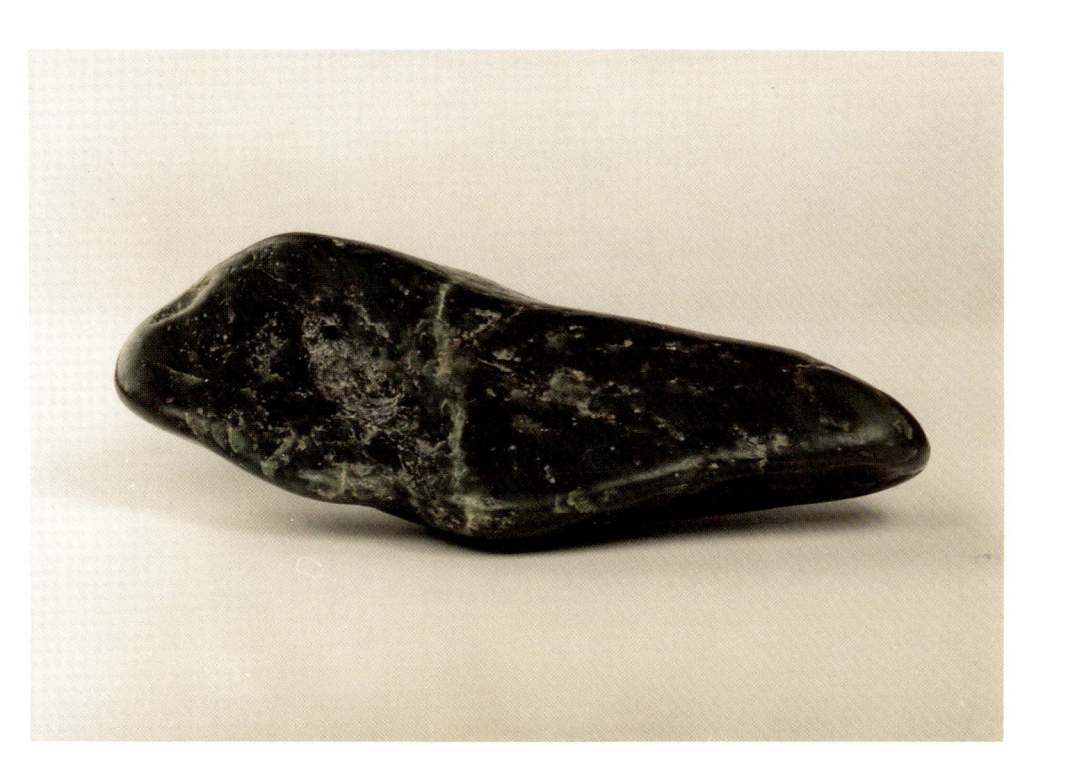

JADITE

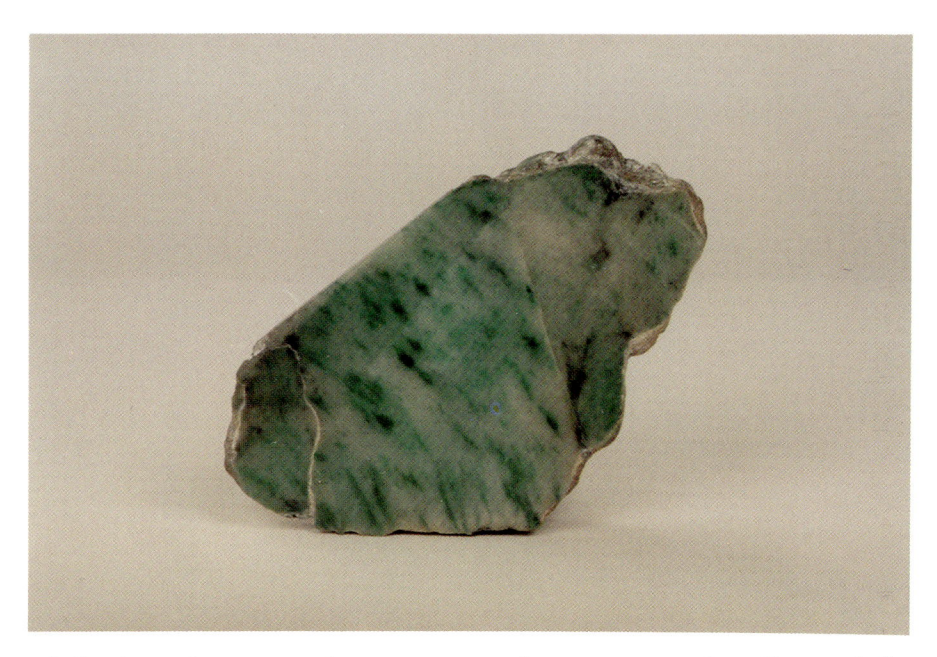

Jadite is semi-opaque and occurs as granular aggregates of small crystals. It may be found in a variety of colors, from yellow to green. Jadite comes principally from Burma, Japan, the United States, and Guatemala.

It is helpful to wear jadite in the form of jewelry, particularly when one is not feeling strong and has to be in large crowds. It will assist in keeping your heart open and will boost your immune system.

HEALING PROPERTIES

CLEANSING AND HEALING FOR THE HEART CHAKRA
STRENGTHENS THE HEART AND KIDNEYS
BOOSTS THE IMMUNE SYSTEM
POWERFUL EMOTIONAL HEALER
DISPELS NEGATIVITY

FOURTH CHAKRA CRYSTAL

KAYANITE

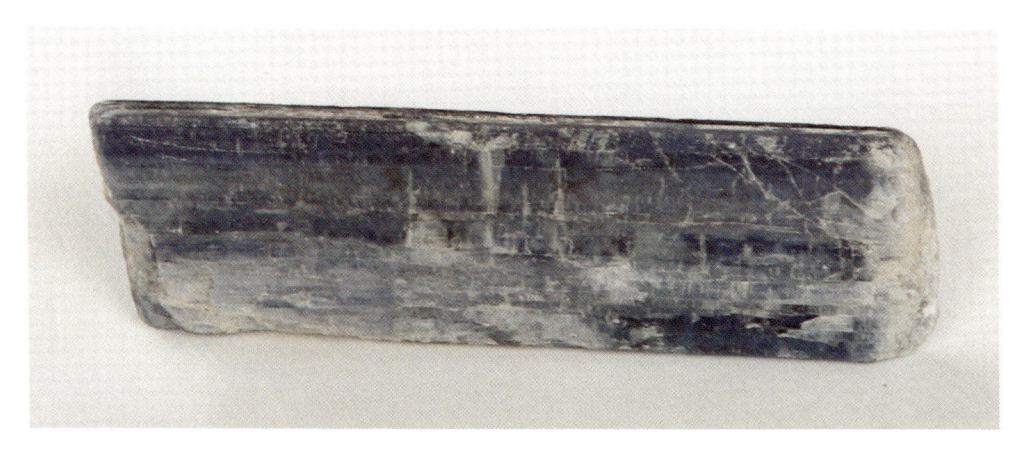

Kayanite has elongated tabular crystals that range from light to dark blue and are rarely terminated. These crystals are found in Switzerland, Italy, Austria, France, Brazil, Kenya, the United States, and India.

This is another of my favorite crystals. I could just melt into the color and stay there. I like to sleep with kayanite under my pillow. I find my dreams take on an expansive tone.

HEALING PROPERTIES

RAISES PHYSICAL VIBRATIONS
CREATES A HIGHER LEVEL OF AWARENESS
STRENGTHENS THE THROAT CHAKRA
AIDS COMMUNICATION WITH THE HIGHER SELF

FIFTH AND SIXTH CHAKRA CRYSTAL

KUNZITE

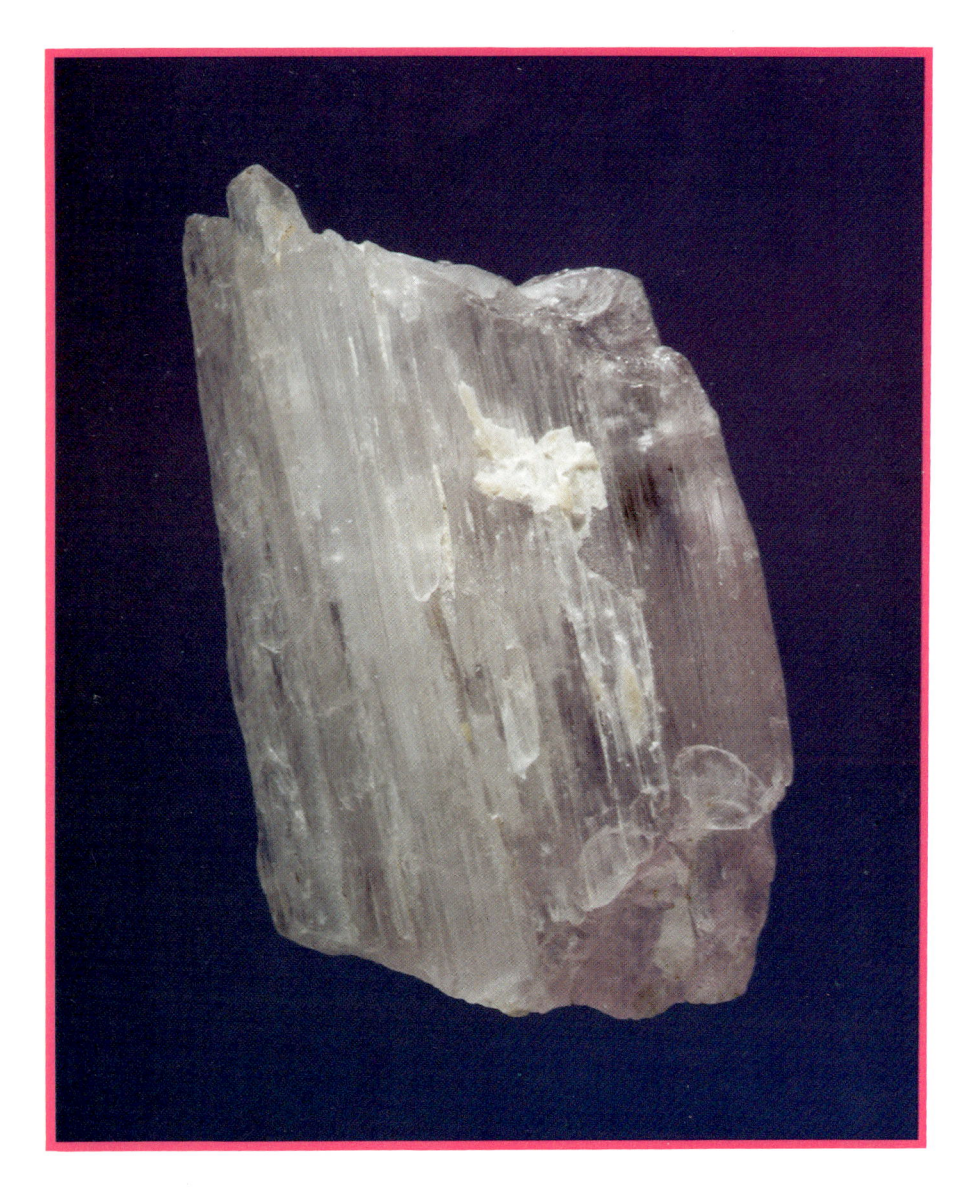

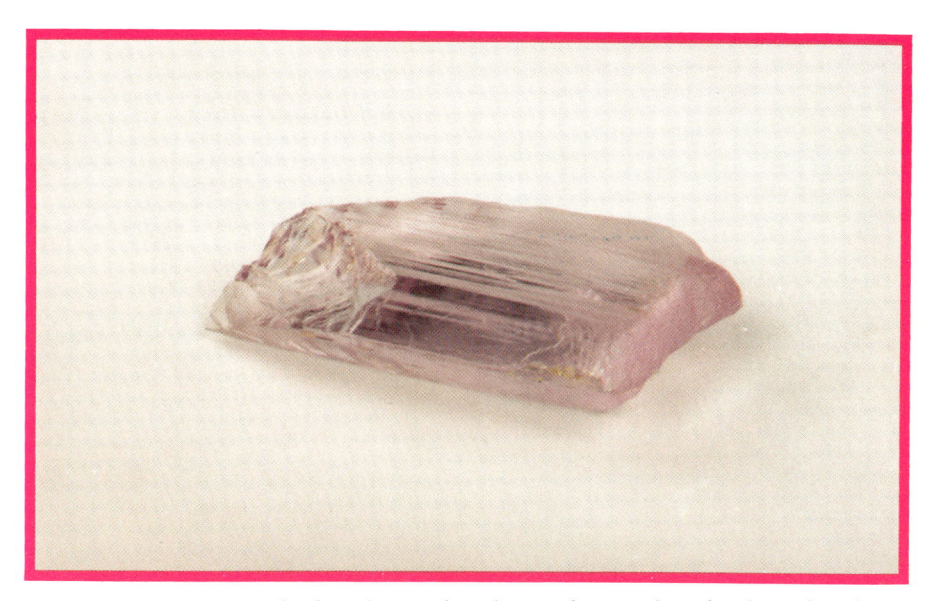

Kunzite is a crystal of violet-pink color and can often be found in large crystals. It is found in the United States, Brazil, and Madagascar.

During a crystal attunement for people who are afraid of love, kunzite placed on the fourth chakra allows the heart to open and receive love.

HEALING PROPERTIES

OPENS THE HEART CHAKRA
HEALS A "BROKEN HEART"
AIDS MANIC DEPRESSION
STRENGTHENS SELF-ESTEEM
OPENS CONNECTION TO HIGHER SELF
STRENGTHENS THE CARDIO-VASCULAR SYSTEM

FOURTH CHAKRA CRYSTAL

LAPIS LAZULI

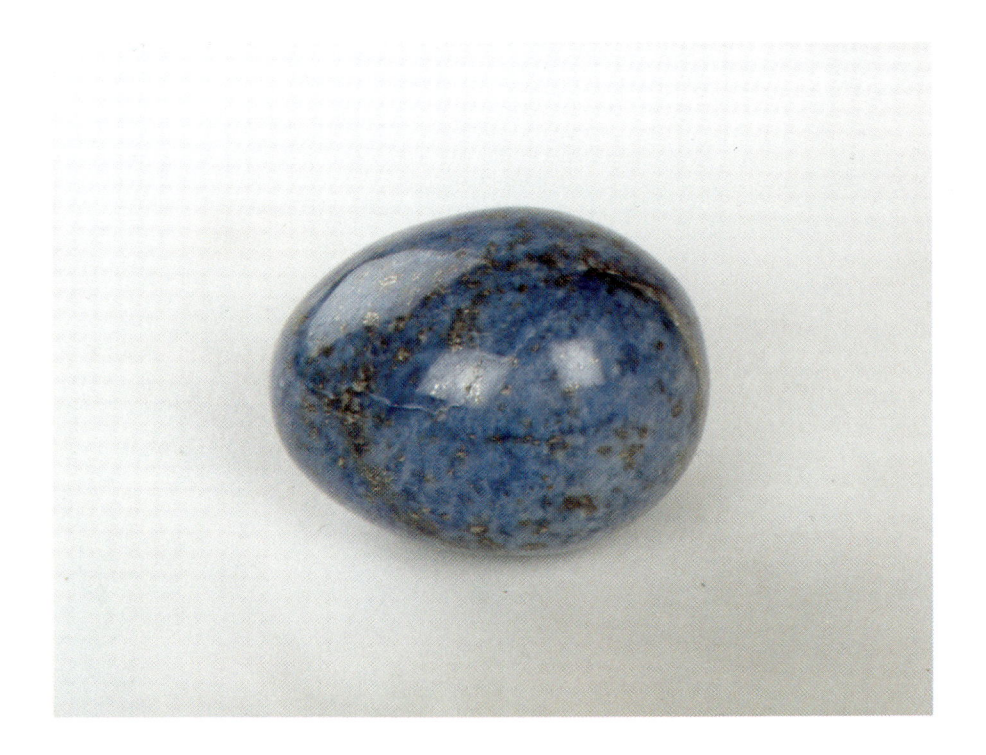

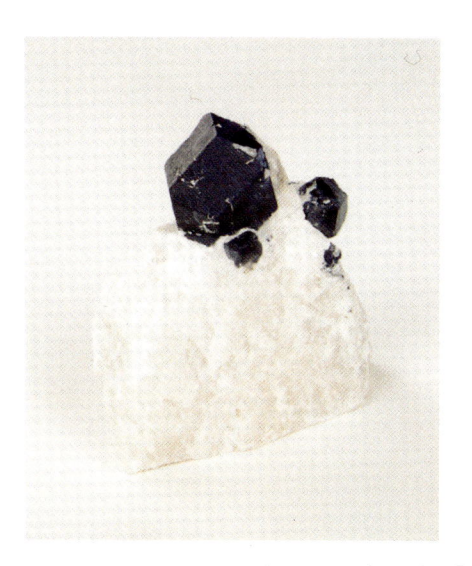

Lapis Lazuli is a semi-opaque stone that is colored a brilliant blue with flecks of pyrite. The most valuable stones are mined in Afghanistan, with smaller quantities coming from the former Soviet Union, Burma, Pakistan, the United States, and Canada.

Lapis Lazuli lends a powerful masculine vibration. Its use as a healing stone dates back to ancient Egypt. In a crystal attunement, lapis used on the fifth chakra helps men feel safe about expressing emotions verbally.

HEALING PROPERTIES

STRENGTHENS THE PHYSICAL BODY
ENHANCES SPIRITUAL AWAKENING
HARMONIZES THE INNER AND OUTER LIFE
ENHANCES PSYCHIC ABILITIES
STRENGTHENS THE SKELETAL SYSTEM
FACILITATES THE OPENING OF ALL CHAKRAS
ACTIVATES THE THYROID
AIDS FERTILITY AND VITALITY
ASSISTS MENTAL CLARITY AND ILLUMINATION

FIFTH AND SIXTH CHAKRA CRYSTAL

MALACHITE

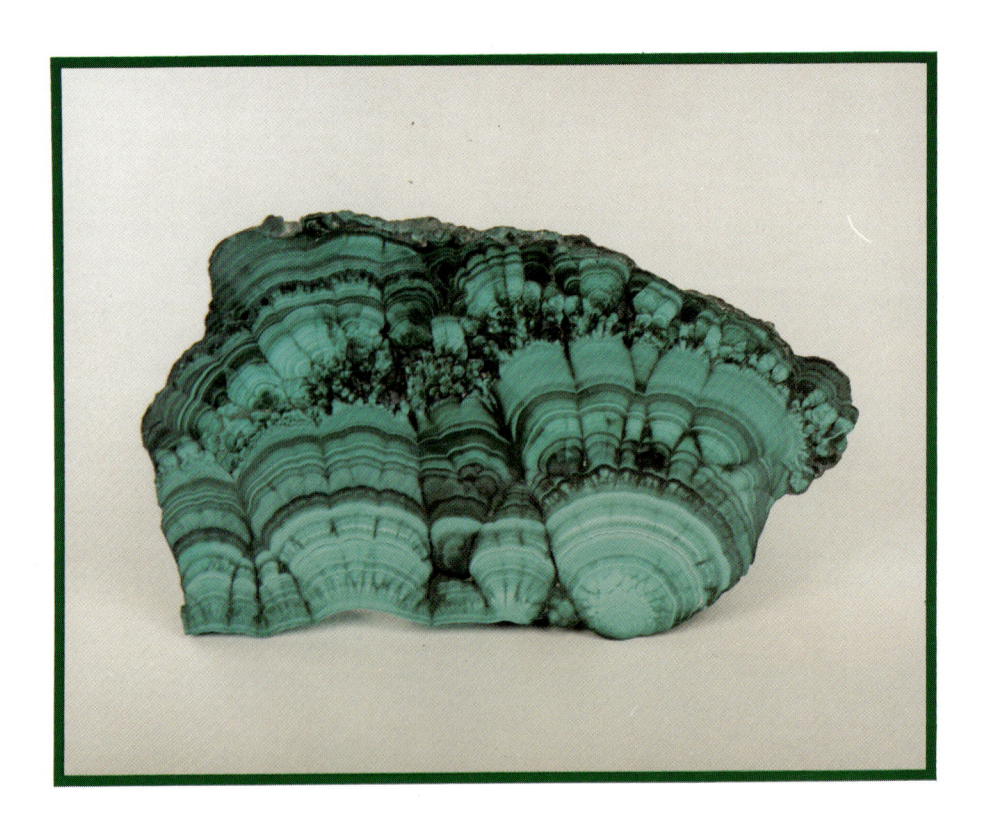

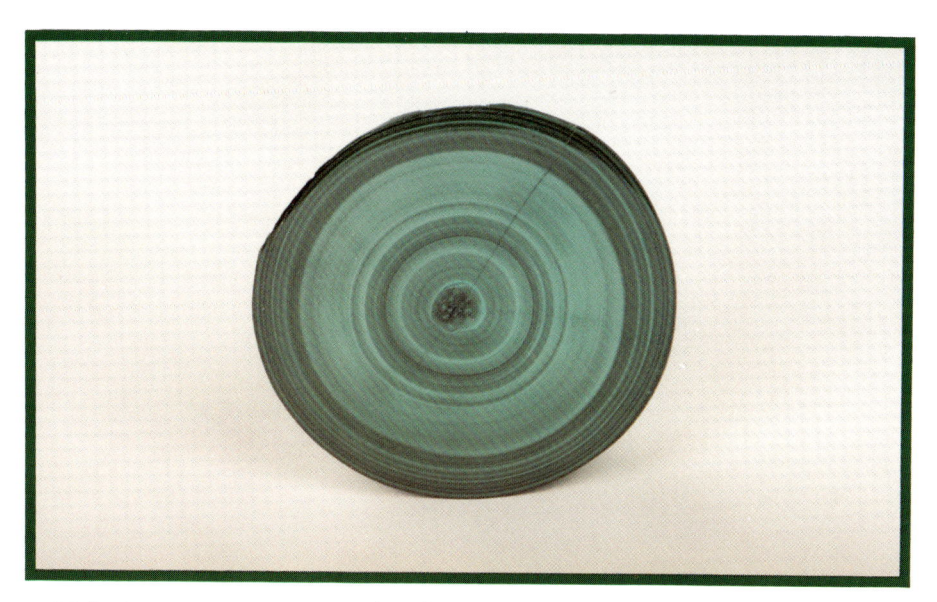

Malachite occurs as circular banded masses consisting of radiating aggregates of elongated crystals. While it is always green in color, it varies from light to dark to black in successive layers of concentration with curvilinear patterns. Large mines are located in the former Soviet Union, Africa, Australia, the United States, Germany, France, and Romania.

If a client comes to me with a problem such as insomnia or nightmares, I recommend placing a piece of malachite at the bedside. Malachite will not only help you sleep, it will bring to your awareness the source of your sleeplessness.

HEALING PROPERTIES

ABSORBS ILLNESSES OF BOTH PHYSICAL AND MENTAL NATURES
AIDS IN THE FUNCTION OF THE PANCREAS AND THE SPLEEN
STRENGTHENS THE HEART AND THE CIRCULATORY SYSTEM
ACTIVATES THE PITUITARY AND THE PINEAL GLAND
USEFUL FOR THE ALLEVIATION OF SLEEP DISORDERS
REVEALS SUBCONSCIOUS BLOCKS

FIFTH AND SIXTH CHAKRA STONE CRYSTAL

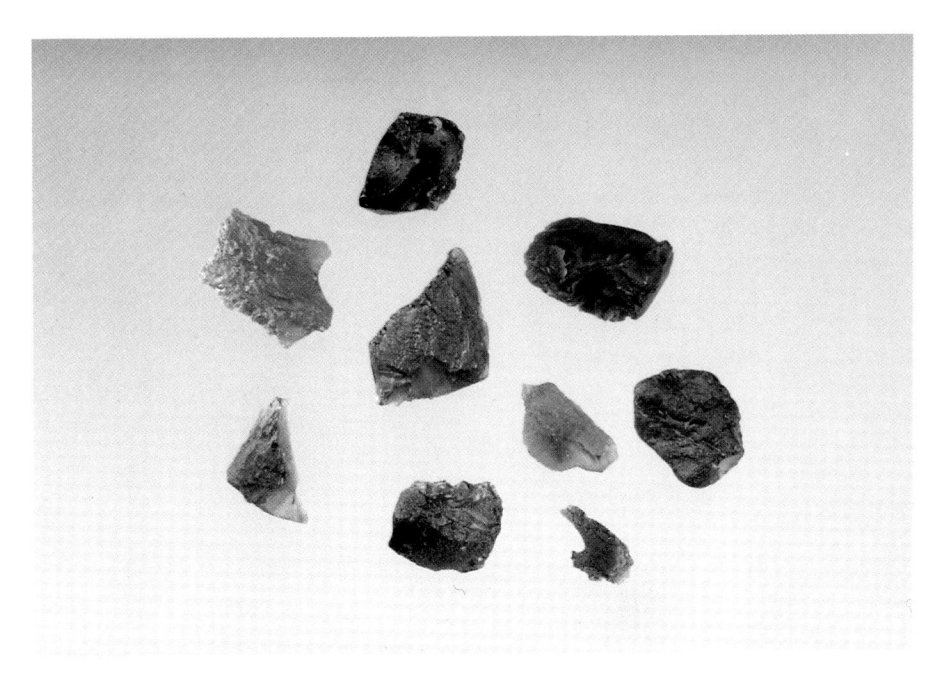

MOLDAVITE

Moldavite is a silica based glassy meteorite with scarred surfaces ranging in color from brown to black to a bottle green.

If it is your desire to expand your psychic abilities I would suggest that you lie down and place moldavite on your sixth chakra. Do this in small increments of time and begin working your way to a total of twenty minutes.

HEALING PROPERTIES

"SEER STONE"
HEALS THE BRAIN AND CENTRAL NERVOUS SYSTEM
HEALS COMA INDUCED BY BODY TRAUMA
AIDS ALIGNMENT WITH THE HIGHER SELF
EXCELLENT AID IN CHANNELING

SIXTH CHAKRA CRYSTAL

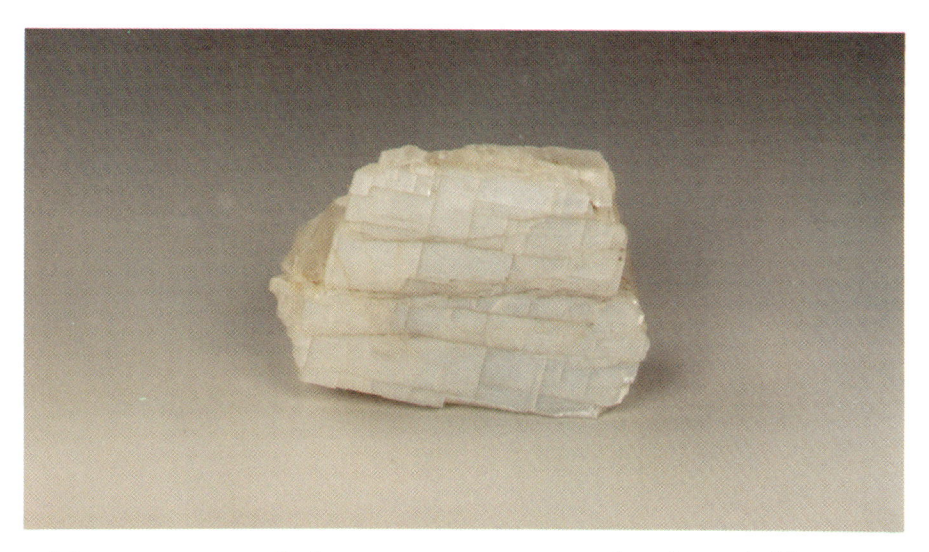

MOONSTONE

Moonstone generally has a transparent ground with a pale blue, gray, yellow, silver, or whitish shimmer. The pale blue type is the most highly prized. This stone is found to occur in Burma, India, Sri Lanka, Australia, Madagascar, the United States and Brazil.

Moonstone is a great stone to carry at a time of menuses or during menopause. Whenever my emotions are running high, I carry moonstones with me.

HEALING PROPERTIES

BALANCES EMOTIONS
UNBLOCKS THE LYMPATHIC SYSTEMS
RELIEVES ANXIETY AND STRESS
USEFUL FOR BALANCING ALL FEMALE PROBLEMS
AIDS IN BIRTHING PROCESS
LESSENS THE TENANCY TO OVERREACT EMOTIONALLY
USEFUL FOR STOMACH, SPLEEN, PANCREAS, AND PITUITARY GLANDS

FOURTH CHAKRA CRYSTAL

OBSIDIAN

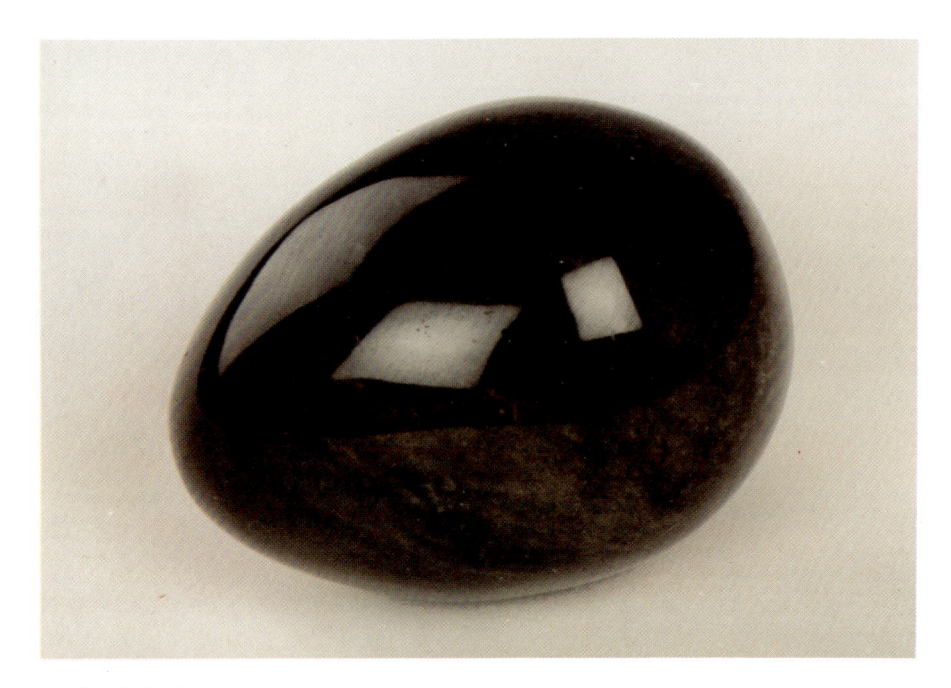

GOLD SHEEN

HEALING PROPERTIES

GROUNDS HIGHER ENERGIES INTO THE PHYSICAL BODY
ACTIVATES THE WILL CENTER
STIMULATES VITALITY

FIRST, THIRD, AND SEVENTH CHAKRA CRYSTAL

BLACK

HEALING PROPERTIES

**PROTECTION FOR SENSITIVE AND PSYCHIC PEOPLE
BALANCES DIGESTIVE AND INTESTINAL SYSTEM
ABSORBS AND DISPERSES NEGATIVITY
STRONG AID FOR CLEARING SUBCONSCIOUS BLOCKS
AIDS DETACHMENT WITH WISDOM AND LOVE
STABILIZES ERRATIC ENERGIES**

FIRST CHAKRA CRYSTAL—ONLY

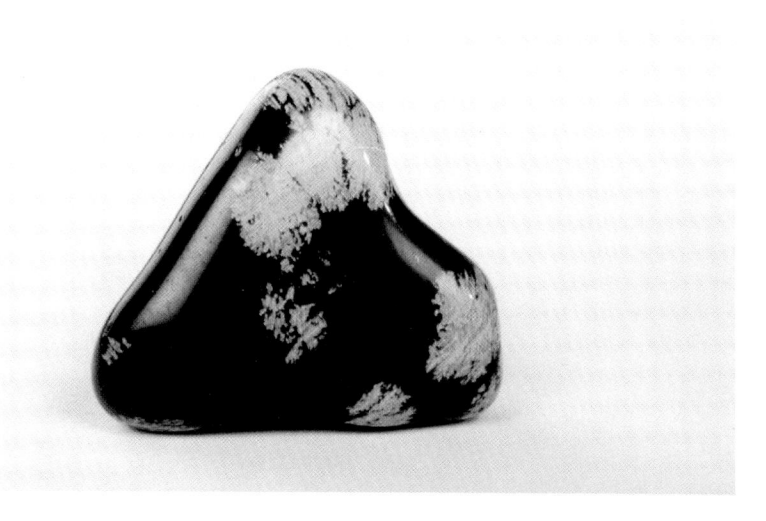

SNOWFLAKE

Obsidian possesses a shiny black color with an obvious glassy texture. Its form occurs from rapidly cooling volcanic magma reaching the earth's surface. This stone is found in Japan, Italy, the United States, and Hungary.

This is a very powerful healing stone; just looking at obsidian can release subconscious blocks. Take care to expect a release when using obsidian on yourself or others.

HEALING PROPERTIES

**ALLOWS FOR A BALANCED ATTITUDE
USEFUL IN MEDITATION, ASTRAL TRAVEL, AND PSYCHIC HEARING
ALLOWS FOR INTEGRATING ALL THE ASPECTS OF ONESELF
PROMOTES TRANSFORMATION**

FIRST CHAKRA CRYSTAL

PERIDOT

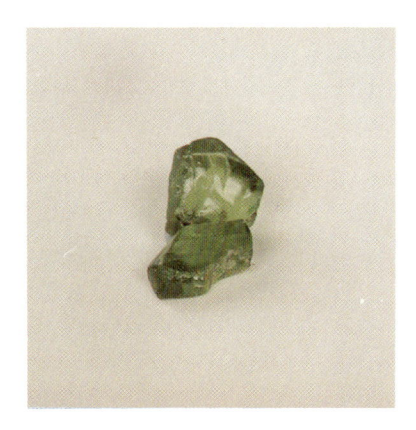

Peridot occurs as a prismatic or anhedral crystal in a yellowish-green to dark green color. The island of Zebirget, in the Red Sea, is an excellent source of this crystal with others coming from the Hawaiian Islands, the United States, Italy and Germany.

The numerous healing properties of peridot and its particularly small size make it a perfect crystal to be worn as jewerly.

HEALING PROPERTIES

STRENGTHENS THE PHYSICAL BODY
STIMULATES AND BALANCES MENTAL PROCESSES
STABILIZES EMOTIONS
ACCELERATES PERSONAL GROWTH
BENEFICIAL ON THE ADRENAL GLANDS
STRENGTHENS HEART, PANCREAS, LIVER AND SPLEEN
REDUCES STRESS IN AN ENVIRONMENT

SECOND, THIRD AND FOURTH

PYRITE

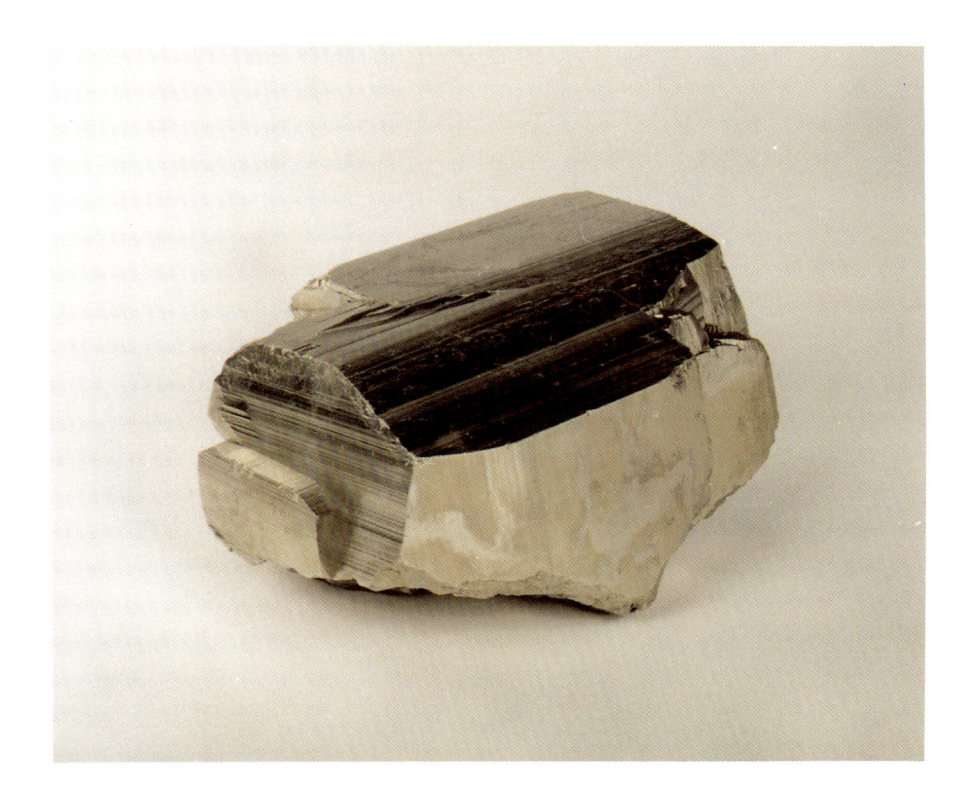

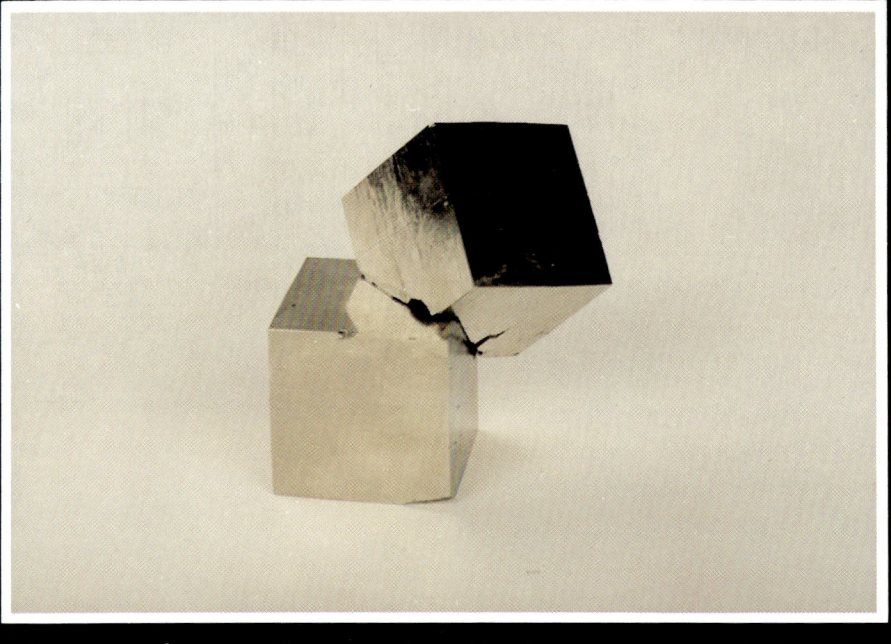

Pyrite is a brassy yellow or pale gold color. It is commonly found in volcanic, sedimentary and metamorphic rocks around the globe and shows up as cubic crystals with striated faces.

Commonly referred to as "fool's gold," this stone is bright and cheery accent that will lift anyones spirits. It is especially good at the bedside of any person who is aged or ill.

HEALING PROPERTIES

WONDERFUL AID IN DIGESTION AND ELIMINATION
INDUCES A POSITIVE OUTLOOK ON LIFE
ENHANCES POWERFUL COMMUNICATION AND INTERACTION
STRENGTHENS PERSONAL WILL

FIRST AND THIRD CHAKRA

QUARTZ

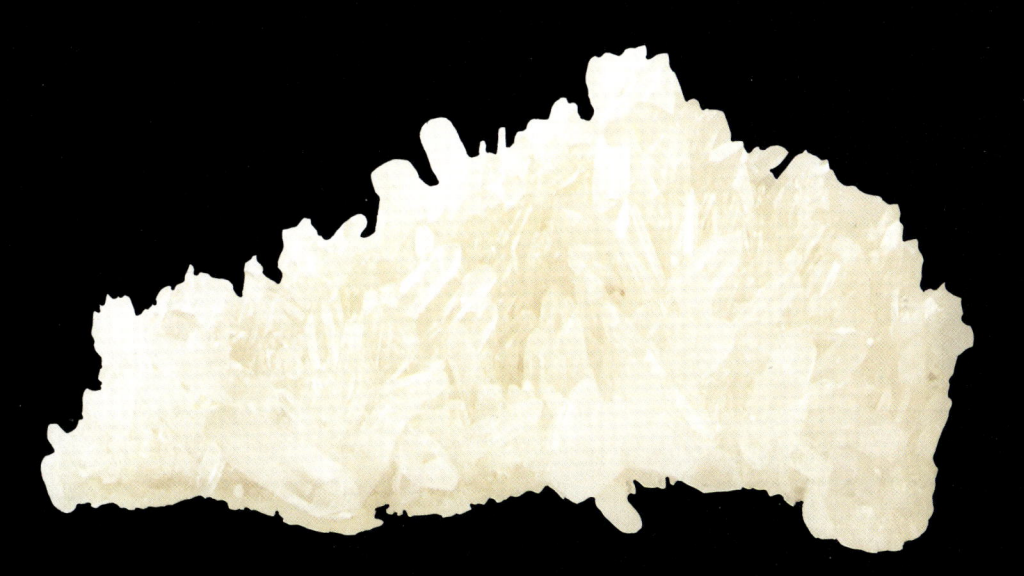

In addition to being described as cryptocrystaline and microcrystalline, quartz occurs in a variety of forms, from well formed crystals to compact masses. Quartz is clear when pure, depending upon the inclusions, it may appear in a rainbow range of colors. This family of crystals occurs worldwide.

TYPES OF QUARTZ

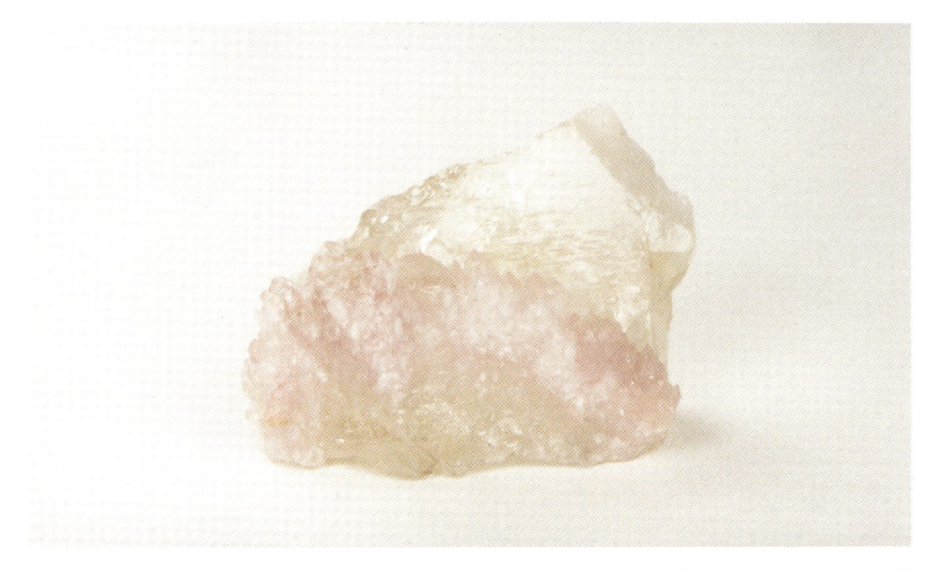

ROSE QUARTZ—The pale pink color is caused by some traces of manganese or titanium in the quartz structure. Well formed crystals are very rare. It is mined in the United States and Brazil.

I always tell clients and friends to place a large piece of rose quartz in their bedroom. This way as you sleep your childhood hurts will be healed. It is also nice to carry a tumbled piece of quartz to strengthen the love vibration.

HEALING PROPERTIES

BALANCING AND CALMING TO THE EMOTIONS
HEALING AID TO THE KIDNEYS
INCREASES FERTILITY
EASES SEXUAL IMBALANCES
HEALING FOR CHILDHOOD TRAUMAS
AIDS IN FORGIVENESS AND COMPASSION

FOURTH CHAKRA CRYSTAL

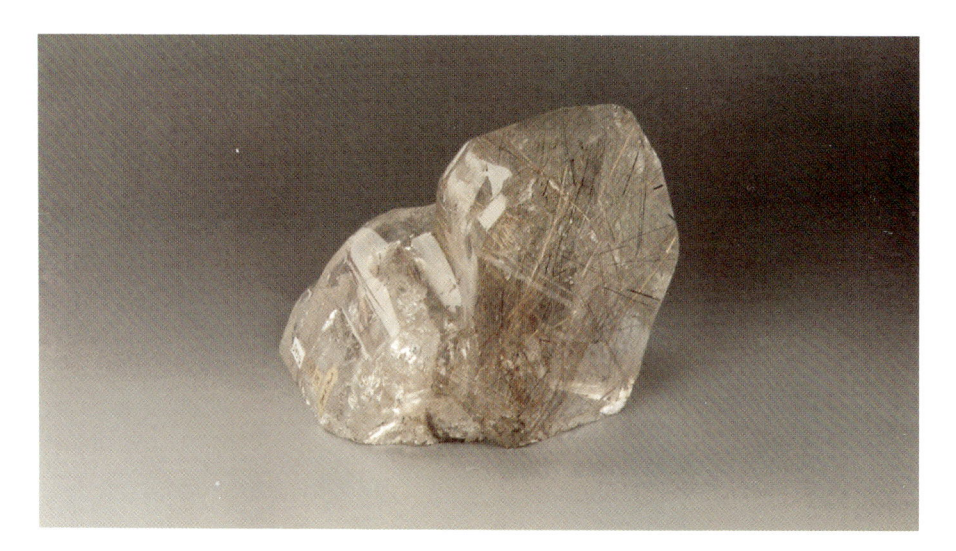

RUTILATED QUARTZ—A well formed clear quartz crystal containing red or yellow rutile, the most famous of which come from Switzerland and Brazil.

Rutilated quartz gives the effective energy boost of a "hot cup of coffee" without the adverse side affects. I recommend you take a few tumbled stones in your pocket when you need a lift.

HEALING PROPERTIES

REGENERATOR—PEOPLE, PLANTS, CRYSTALS, AND ANIMALS
HELPS RESIST AGING
STRENGTHENS THE IMMUNE SYSTEM
EASES DEPRESSION
TRANSMUTES NEGATIVITY
ENHANCES THE ABILITY TO COMMUNICATE WITH ONE'S HIGHER SELF

ALL CHAKRA CRYSTAL

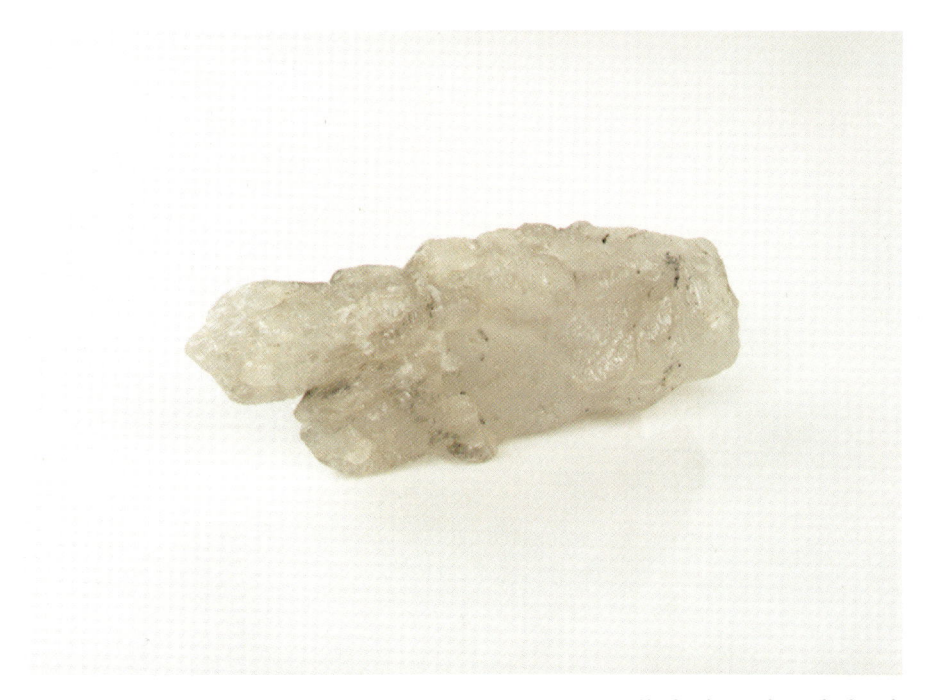

SKELETAL QUARTZ—These are sometimes called elestials. Skeletal quartz resembles smokey quartz in appearance with very distinct etched patterns on the surface. They are often found in or close to water, possibly with water inclusions.

A crystal attunement that will significantly raise your vibration is to place skeletal quartz on each of your seven chakras for twenty minutes.

HEALING PROPERTIES

AIDS IN RAISING SUBCONSCIOUS THOUGHTS
AMPLIFIES AND MAGNIFIES EMOTIONS
EXTREMELY POWERFUL AND BLUNT IN WHAT IS REVEALED
STRONG CONNECTION TO THE ANGELIC KINGDOM

ALL CHAKRA CRYSTAL

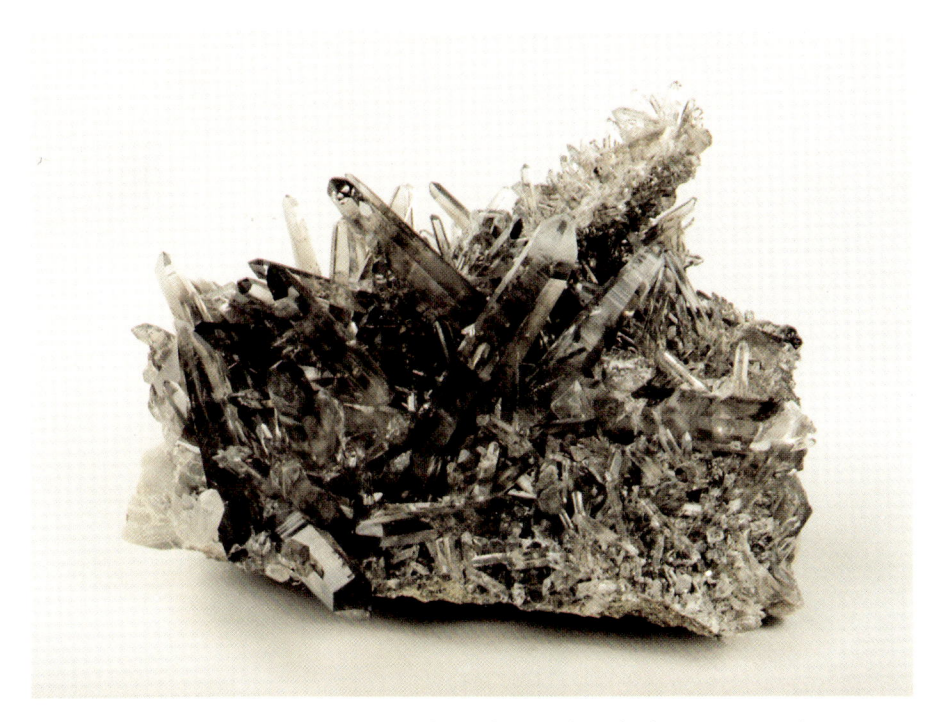

SMOKEY QUARTZ—Clear and smokey colored, this variety of quartz is said to be caused when naturally exposed to radioactivity. This crystal is found most often in hydro—thermal veins in Brazil and Scotland.

When I do a crystal attunement I usually put smokey quartz on the first chakra. This is an effective way to help pull the vibrations of the other stones into the body.

HEALING PROPERTIES

STIMULATES THE ADRENAL GLANDS
GROUNDS SPIRITUAL ENERGY INTO THE PHYSICAL BODY
AID IN CASES OF DEPRESSION
GROUNDING

FIRST CHAKRA CRYSTAL

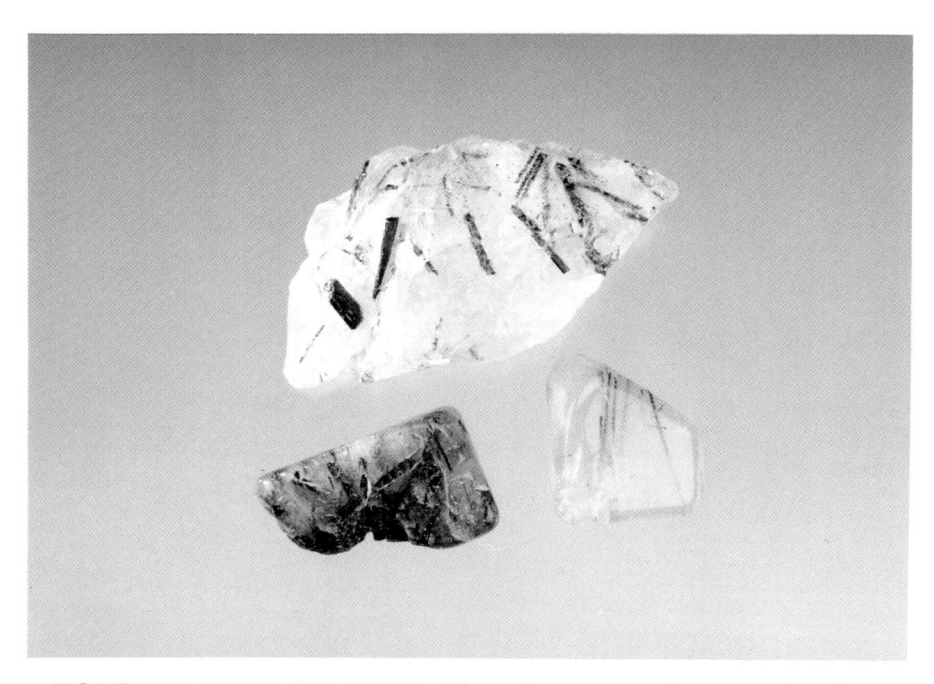

TOURMALATED QUARTZ—This clear crystal quartz has black tourmaline inclusions. Brazil and Sri Lanka are the primary sources of tourmalated quartz.

If you are easily influenced by circumstances or people around you, make it a habit to carry tourmalated quartz or wear it as an item of jewelry. This vibration will keep you distinct from the people and circumstances around you.

HEALING PROPERTIES

BALANCES MALE AND FEMALE POLARITIES
VERY STRONG GROUNDING
GOOD PSYCHIC PROTECTION FROM AGGRESSIVE ENERGIES

ALL CHAKRA CRYSTAL

RHODOCHROSITE

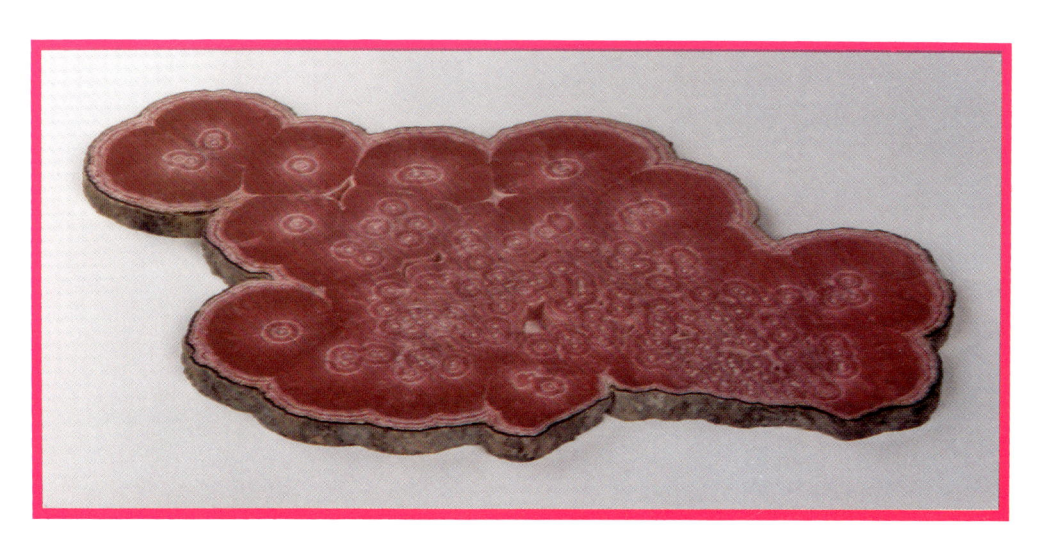

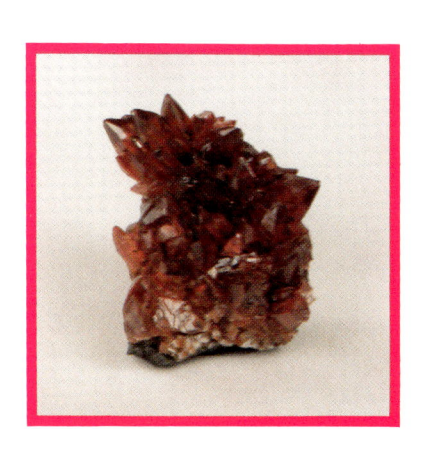

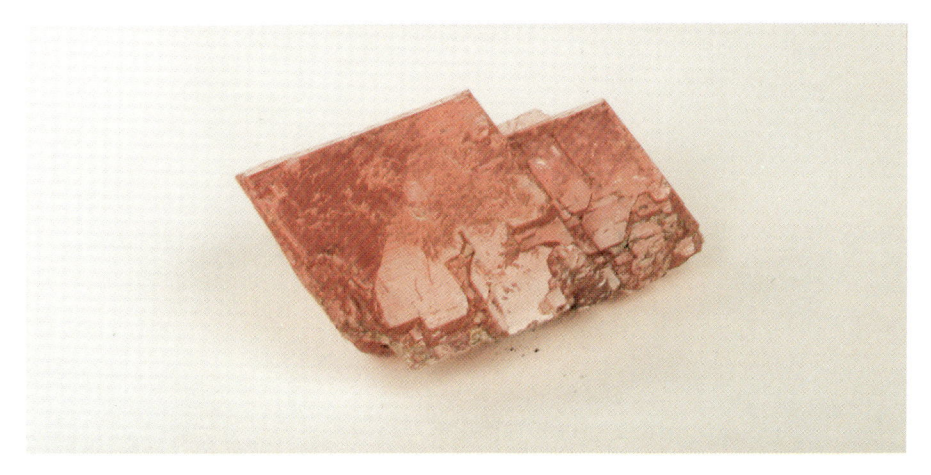

Rhodochrosite is a bright pink crystal most commonly formed in banded stalactic masses. It is mined in Romania, South America, the United States, Argentina, Mexico, Germany, and Italy.

When I am doing a crystal attunement on a woman, I always put rhodochrosite on the second chakra. We all have issues with our feminity and this is the perfect vibration to heal them.

HEALING PROPERTIES

ENHANCES MEMORY AND THE INTELLECT
HEALS EMOTIONAL WOUNDS
BRINGS LOVE INTO THE LOWER CHAKRAS
AIDS IN SELF ACCEPTANCE AND FORGIVENESS
USEFUL IN HEALING RAPE AND INCEST TRAUMA

FIRST, SECOND, AND THIRD CHAKRA CRYSTAL

RUBY

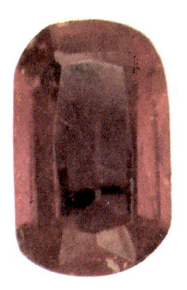

Ruby is the most valuable variety of corundum and known for its red hues. The most famous rubies come from Burma with others coming from Thailand, Sri Lanka, India, and Pakistan.

Although ruby is a first chakra crystal and a passionate color, it has a distinctly spiritual vibration. This is a good stone for raising sexual energies to a higher expression of consciousness.

HEALING PROPERTIES

HIGH ENERGY BOOST
INCREASES PERSONAL COURAGE
AIDS EMOTIONAL AND PHYSICAL STABILITY
STRENGTHENS IMMUNITY
ALLOWS SELFLESS SERVICE AND SPIRITUAL DEVOTION

FIRST AND FOURTH CHAKRA

SAPPHIRE

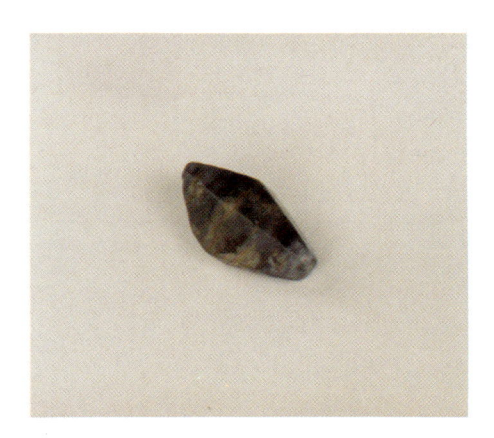

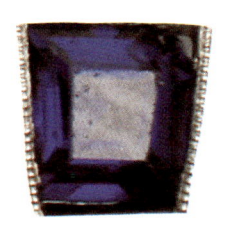

Sapphire is a variety of corundum which runs the rainbow spectrum of colors. The finest sapphire comes from Kashmir, Burma, Sri Lanka, and Thailand.

As far as healing stones go, the quality or grade of the particular stone is relatively unimportant. It is the color and vibration that we are concerned with when choosing a healing stone. A sapphire does not have to be gem quality to be an effective healing crystal.

HEALING PROPERTIES

BLUE SAPPHIRE
ENHANCES INTUITION
CALMS THE MIND
AIDS THE DIGESTIVE SYSTEM
MILDLY GROUNDING

FIRST AND SIXTH CHAKRA CRYSTAL

SELENITE

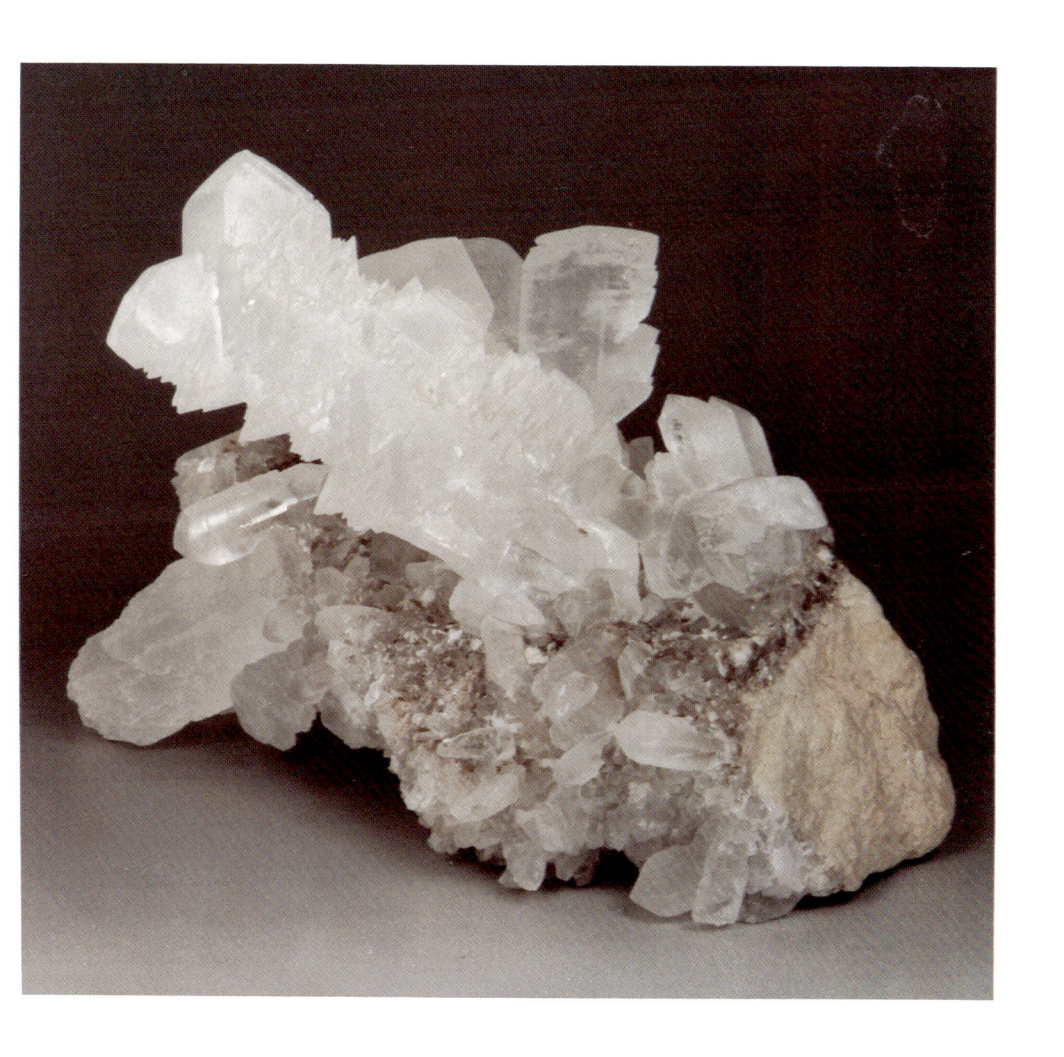

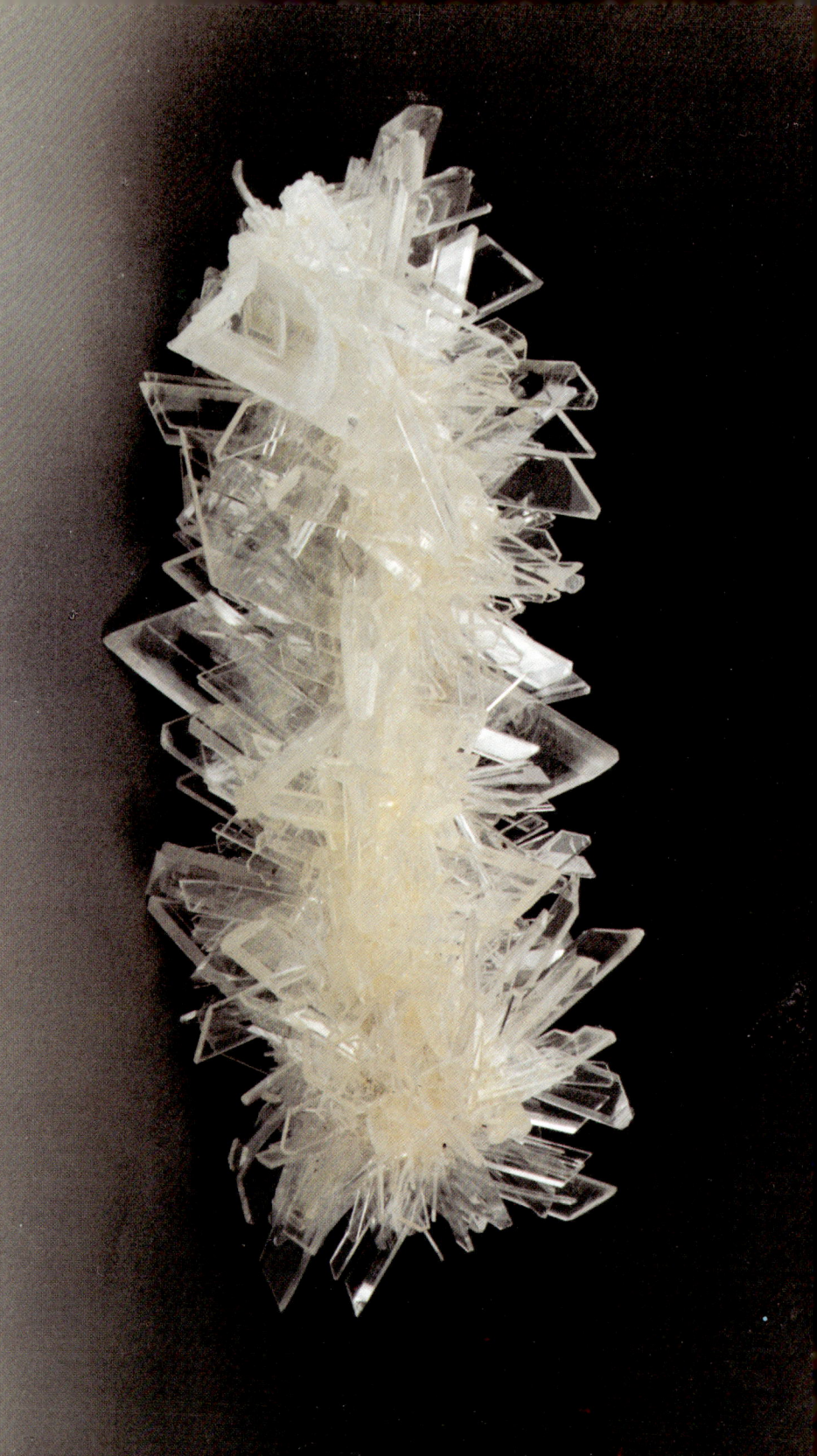

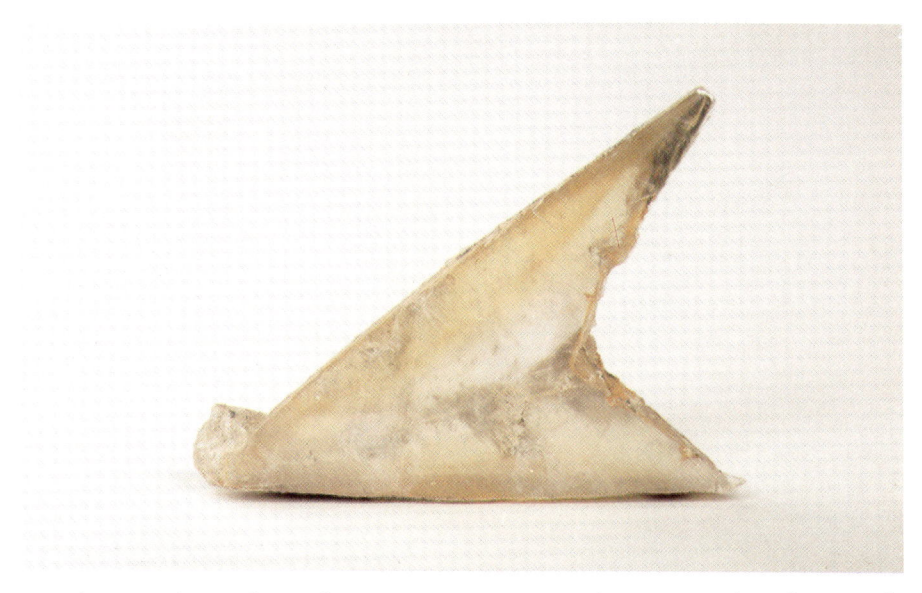

Selenite is formed, as salt water evaporates, in clear, striated, and very soft crystal. It is commonly found throughout the world. Selenite formations are arrowhead, desert rose, fish tail and floret.

A soft and feminine vibration that lends the experience of safety in feminity. This is a great stone for women to carry who find it fearful and unsafe to be soft.

HEALING PROPERTIES

LENDS MENTAL AND SPIRITUAL EXPANSION
SOOTHES THE NERVOUS SYSTEM
STRENGTHENS WILL POWER

SEVENTH CHAKRA CRYSTAL

SODOLITE

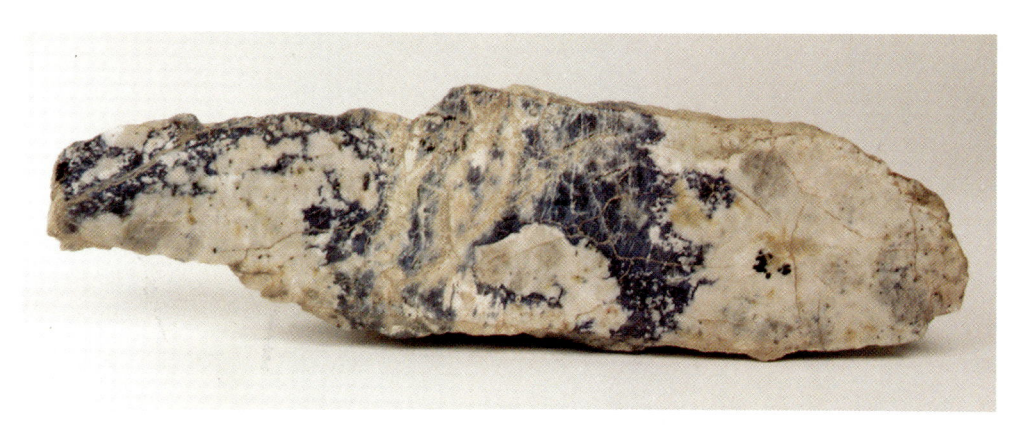

Sodolite is usually found in compact masses. It is bright blue in color with white or gray streaks throughout. The United States is the primary location for sodolite deposits, although it has been found in Canada, Brazil, Greenland, Romania, Portugal, Burma, the former Soviet Union, and Italy.

This stone gets people talking. If you have a friend who just will not open up, try giving them a piece of Sodolite to carry around.

HEALING PROPERTIES

BALANCES THE ENDOCRINE SYSTEM
STRENGTHENS THE LYMPHATIC SYSTEM
REDUCES FEARS AND GUILTS
AIDS IN COMMUNICATION AND SELF EXPRESSION
VERY GROUNDING

FIFTH AND SIXTH CHAKRA

SULFUR

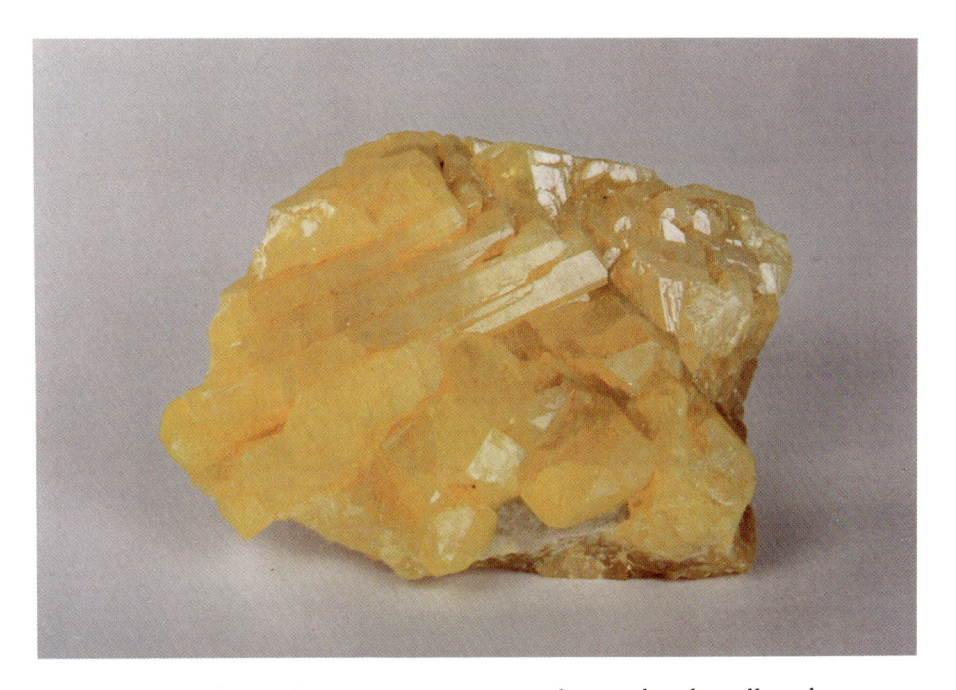

Sulfur crystals may be transparent to translucent, bright yellow, brown or black. The finest sulfur crystals come from Italy and Japan.

In crystalline form sulfur is one of the most beautiful minerals. The bright yellow sulfur crystals give off a vitality that is surpassed only by the golden light of the sun.

HEALING PROPERTIES

ENHANCES PHYSICAL STRENGTH
LENDS VITALITY
STRENGTHENS AND HEALS THE WILL CENTER

THIRD CHAKRA CRYSTAL

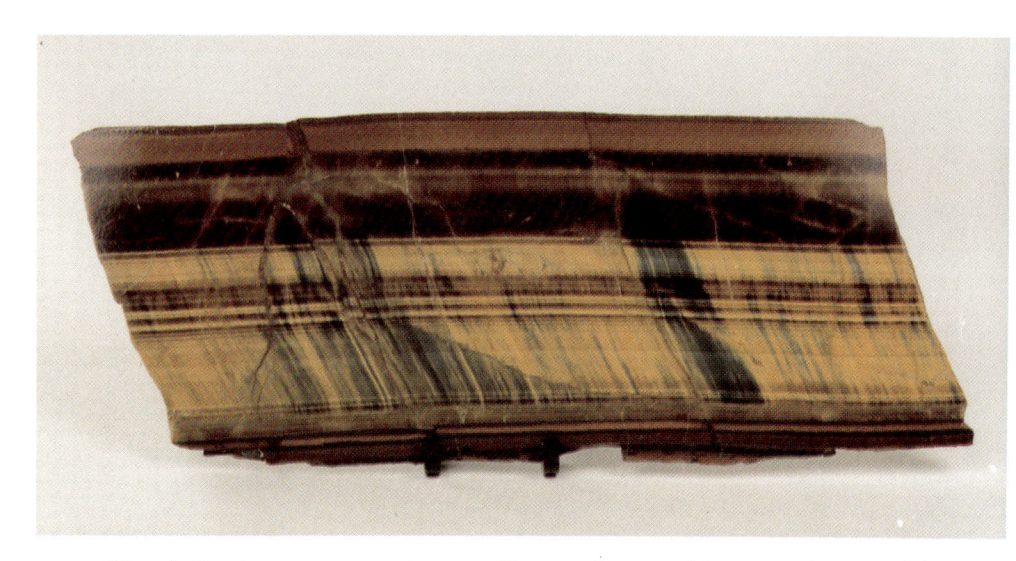

TIGER'S EYE

Tiger's Eye is quartz containing yellow and brown fibrous inclusions. This variety of quartz comes principally from South Africa.

Are you stubborn, or do you know someone who is? Tiger's Eye is the solution. The vibration is flow, and flow they will, with a tiger's eye pendant or ring.

HEALING PROPERTIES

FLOW IN COMMUNICATION
USEFUL TO GAIN INSIGHT INTO ANY AREA
BENEFICIAL TO SPLEEN, PANCREAS, DIGESTIVE SYSTEM AND COLON
HELPS SOFTEN STUBBORNNESS
GOOD GROUNDING STONE

THIRD CHAKRA CRYSTAL

TOPAZ

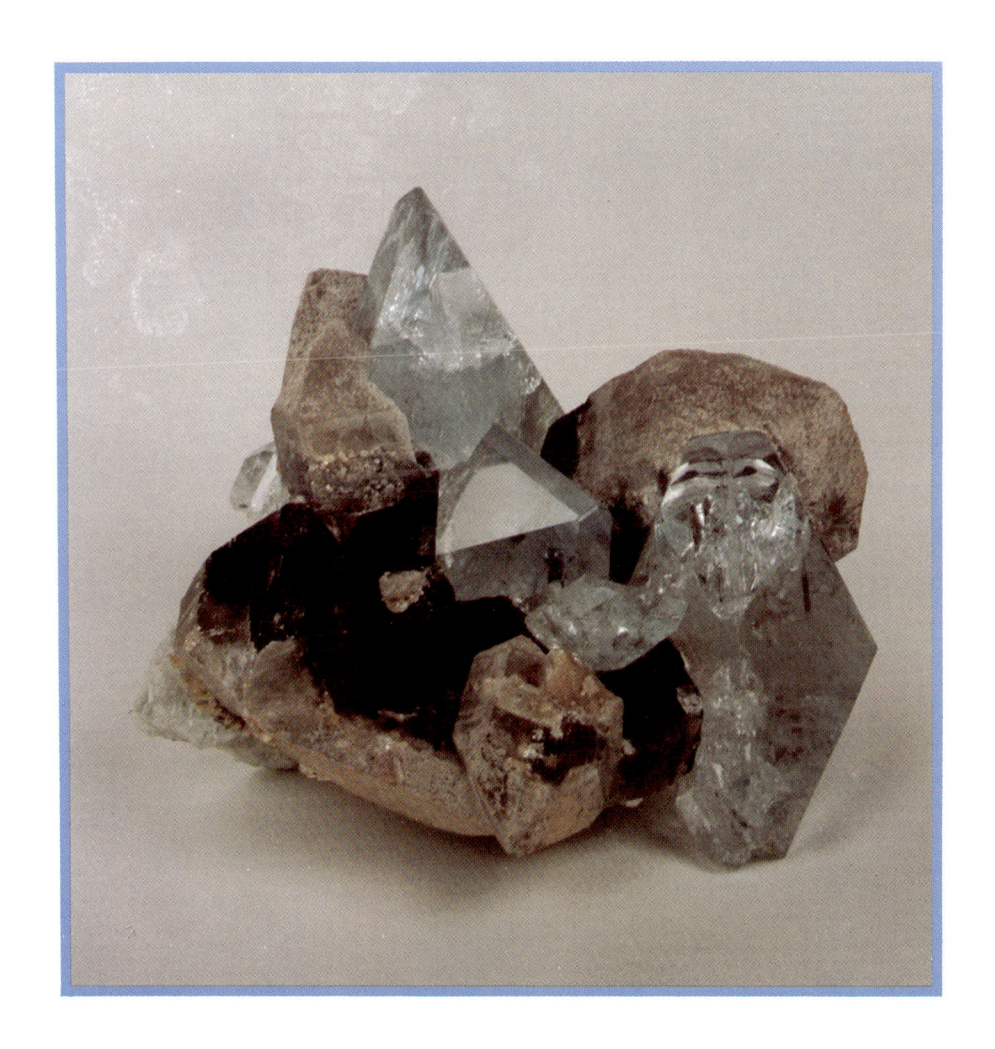

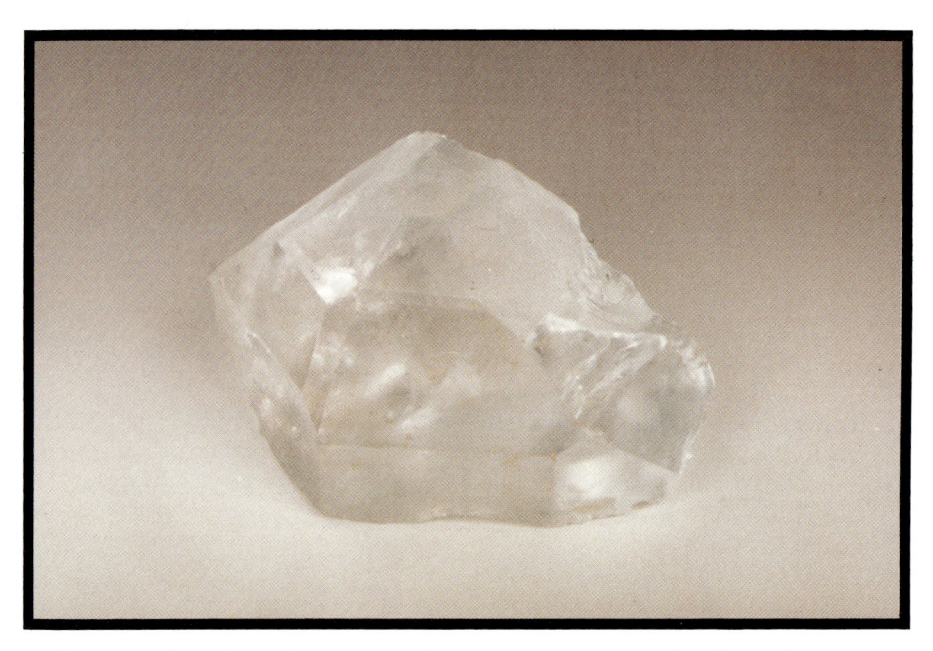

Topaz is often found in short or long prismatic crystals. The color ranges vary from a soft yellow honey to golden brown and blue to pink. Brazil claims the most beautiful crystals in the world. Topaz is also found in Mexico, the United States, Sri Lanka, Japan, the former Soviet Union, and Africa.

Some people swear by copper for the relief of arthritis. I swear by topaz. Try it and see if it works for you. You can find a relatively inexpensive piece at your local New Age bookstore or crystal shop.

HEALING PROPERTIES

**VERY HELPFUL FOR THE DIGESTIVE SYSTEM
OPENS THE CROWN CHAKRA
USEFUL IN REGENERATING TISSUE
STRENGTHENING LIVER, GALL BLADDER AND SPLEEN
RELIEVES DEPRESSION, ANGER AND FEAR
HELPFUL IN RELIEVING ARTHRITIS AND RHEUMATISM**

THIRD AND SEVEN CHAKRA CRYSTALS

TOURMALINE

Tourmaline has elongated prismatic crystals with vertical striations that occur in forms transparent to opaque. The finest tourmaline can be found in Italy, Brazil, the former Soviet Union, Africa, and the United States.

I believe tourmaline, in all it's colors, to be the most useful and beautiful of the new age healing stones. A full body attunement using all the colors of tourmaline is a wonderful treat for raising vibrational frequencies.

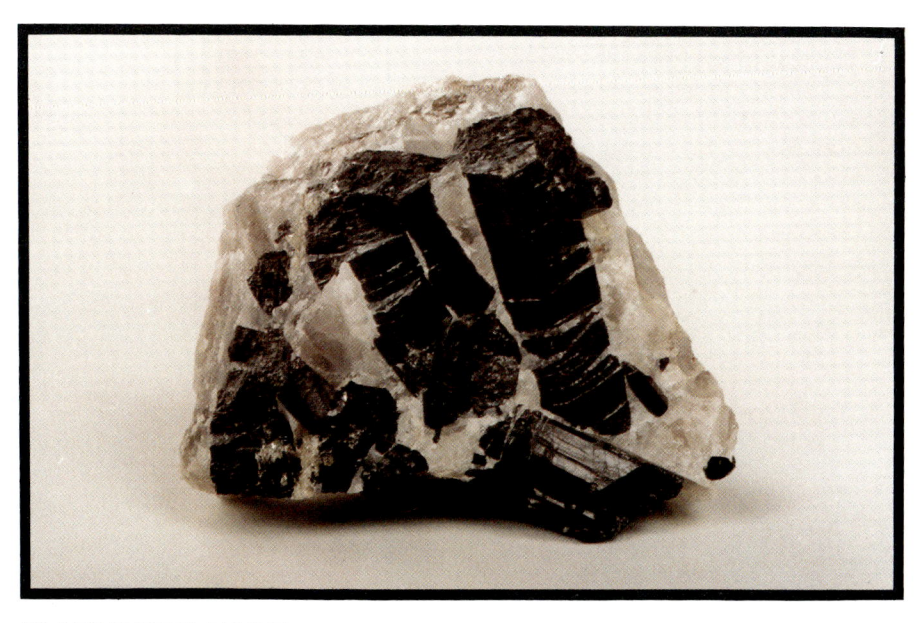

BLACK TOURMALINE

HEALING PROPERTIES

**LENDS PSYCHIC PROTECTION FROM NEGATIVE INFLUENCES
GROUNDS SPIRITUAL ENERGIES INTO THE BODY
VERY GROUNDING**

FIRST CHAKRA CRYSTAL

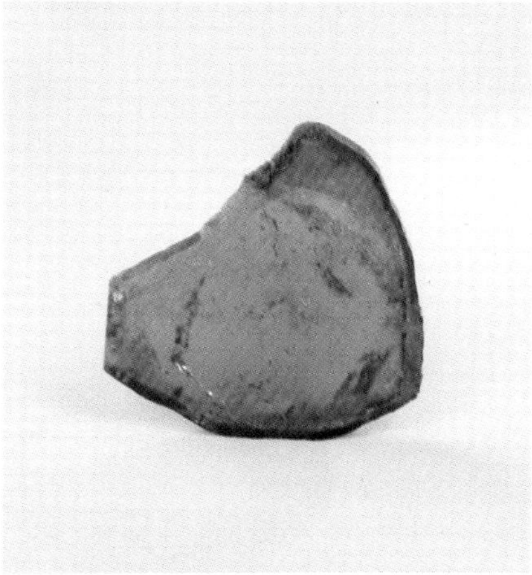

BLUE TOURMALINE

HEALING PROPERTIES

**LENDS INNER PEACE
CALMS ANGER AND FRUSTRATION
RELIEVES SADNESS
ENABLES CLEAR VISUAL PERCEPTION
HEALS SORE THROATS
AIDS THYROID GLAND**

FIFTH CHAKRA CRYSTAL

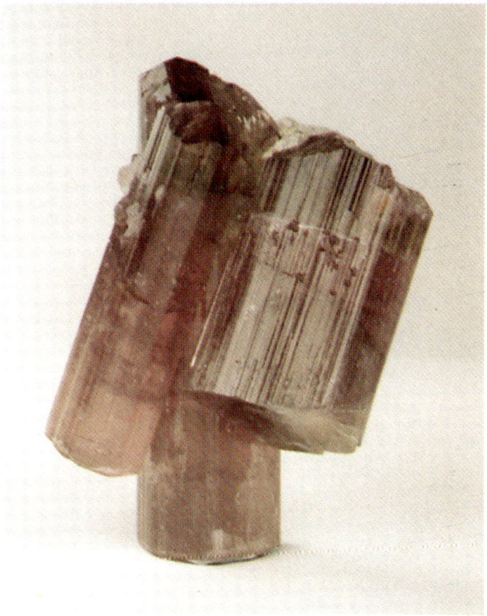

PINK/RED TOURMALINE

HEALING PROPERTIES

PROMOTES THE ATTITUDE OF BEING YOUNG AT HEART
CREATES THE READINESS FOR OUTWARD EXPRESSION
HEALS FEAR AND NEGATIVITY HELD IN THE HEART
STRONG INFUSION OF THE LOVE VIBRATION
ACTIVATES LOVE AND DEVOTION
STIMULATES GROUNDED PASSION

FOURTH CHAKRA CRYSTAL

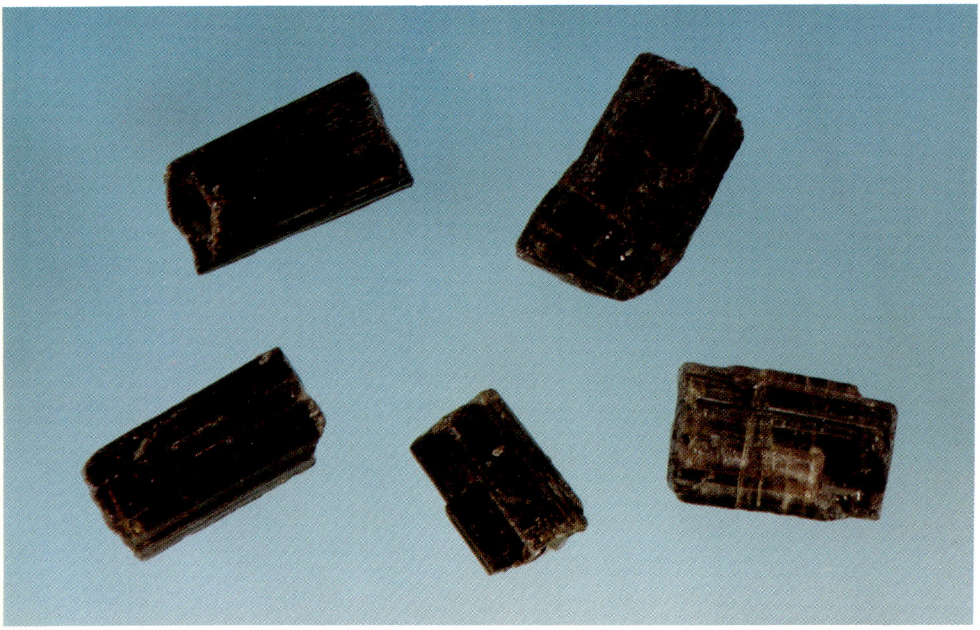

GREEN TOURMALINE

HEALING PROPERTIES

**BENEFICIAL FOR HEALING THE ENDOCRINE SYSTEM
EXCELLENT ANTIDEPRESSANT
ENHANCES SENSITIVITY AND UNDERSTANDING**

FOURTH CHAKRA CRYSTAL

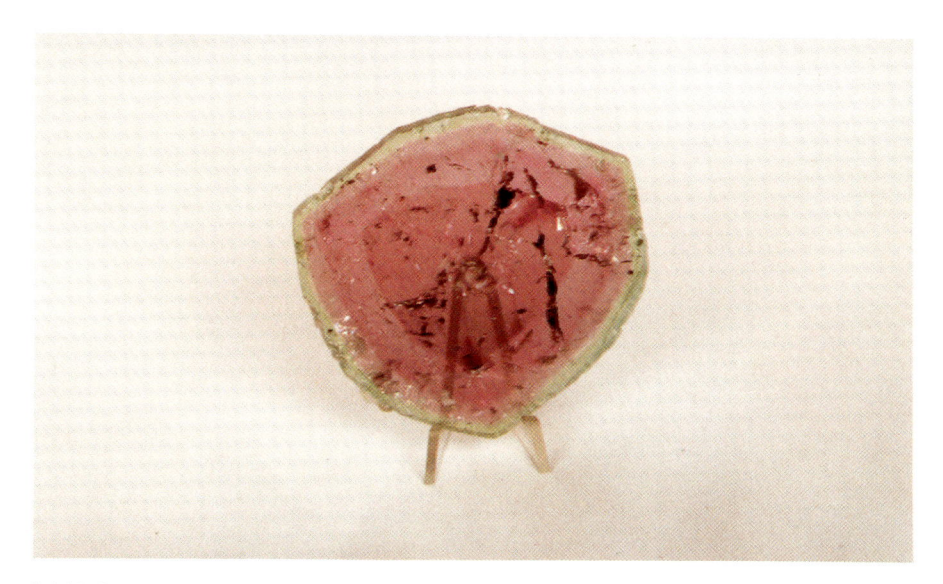

WATERMELON TOURMALINE

HEALING PROPERTIES

**GROUNDS THE HEALING LOVE VIBRATION INTO THE BODY
RELEASES EMOTIONAL PAIN
HEALS A "BROKEN HEART"**

FIRST AND FOURTH CHAKRA CRYSTALS

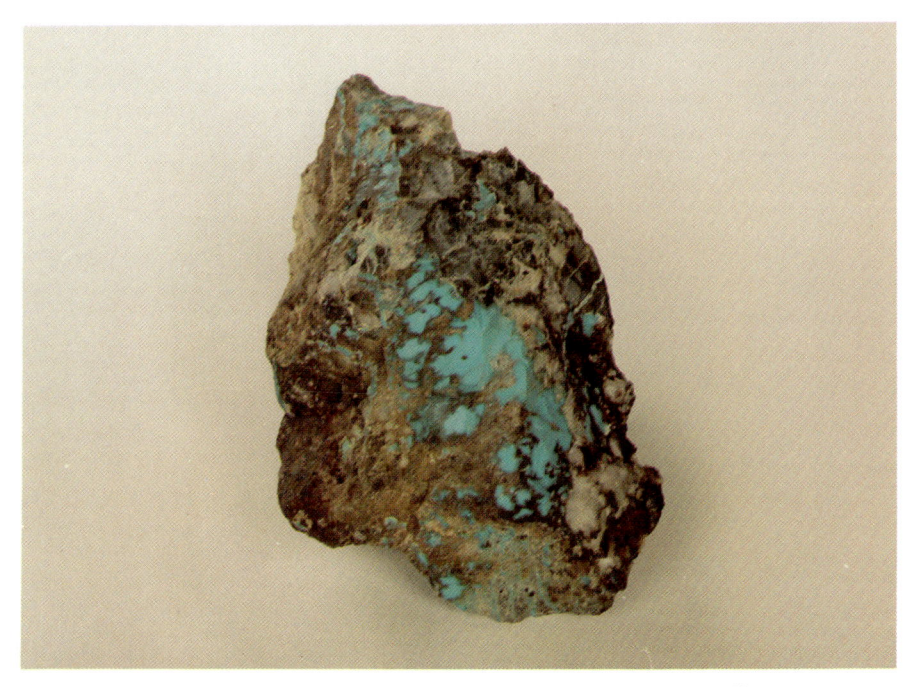

TURQUOISE

Turquoise usually occurs in green or pale blue microcrystalline masses or veins. The most coveted pale blue variety comes from Iran or Egypt with those from the United States being less popular because of their greenish hue.

The healing properties make turquoise appropriate as an object of adornment. On those days when you need to balance your vibrations, this stone helps to balance all your chakras.

HEALING PROPERTIES

STRENGTHENS THE ENTIRE BODY
OPENS ALL THE CHAKRAS
GREAT AID TO COMMUNICATION
LENDS VITALITY TO THE NERVOUS SYSTEM
CALMING EFFECT TO THE EMOTIONAL BODY

FOURTH AND FIFTH CHAKRA STONES

CHAPTER TWO

CROSS REFERENCES

CRYSTALS SHOULD BE USED IN CONJUNCTION WITH TRADITIONAL MEDICAL THERAPIES.
CRYSTALS AND STONES THAT RELATE TO SPECIFIC BODY PARTS AND DISORDERS

ABSORBS ILLNESS
BLOODSTONE
CLEAR QUARTZ
MALACHITE

ABUSE ISSUES
MOONSTONE
RHODOCHROSITE

ADRENAL GLANDS
PERIDOT
SMOKEY QUARTZ

ARTHRITIS
FLORITE
TOPAZ

BALANCES CHAKRAS
TURQUOISE
CHRYSOCOLLA

BLOOD DISORDERS
AVENTURINE
BLOODSTONE
GARNET/RED

COLON
CITRINE
OBSIDIAN/BLACK

DEPRESSION
KUNZITE
QUARTZ/RUTILATED
QUARTZ/SMOKEY
QUARTZ
TOPAZ

EYE STRAIN
CALCITE/TRANSPARENT
EMERALDS

FEAR ISSUES
AQUAMARINE
CHRYSOCOLLA
SODOLITE
TOPAZ

FEMALE ISSUES
CHRYSOCOLLA
MOONSTONE
RHODOCHROSITE

FERTILITY
LAPIS LAZULI
QUARTZ/ROSE

FLUID RETENTION
AQUAMARINE

GROUNDING
BLOODSTONE
FLORITE/ALL COLORS
HEMATITE
QUARTZ/SMOKEY
QUARTZ/TOURMALATED
SODOLITE
TOURMALINE/BLACK
TOURMALINE/GREEN
TIGER'S EYE

GALL BLADDER
CITRINE
TOPAZ

HEART/CARDIO-VASCULAR
BLOODSTONE
FLORITE
JADE
KUNZITE
MALACHITE
PERIDOT
TOURMALINE/GREEN

HYPER-ACTIVITY
QUARTZ/TOURMALATED

IMMUNE SYSTEM
CITRINE
EMERALD
JADE
QUARTZ/RUTILATED
RUBY

INFECTIONS
AGATE/BLUE LACE

KIDNEY
CITRINE
JADE
QUARTZ/ROSE

KUNDALINE
BLOODSTONE
GARNET/RED

LIVER
CITRINE
PERIDOT
TOPAZ

LUNGS/RESPIRATORY SYSTEM
CHRYSOCOLLA
TURQUOISE

LYMPH SYSTEM
AGATE/BLUE LACE
SODOLITE

MENTAL PROCESSES
AGATE/BLUE LACE
AMETHYST
AQUAMARINE
AZURITE
CALCITE/GREEN
CELESTITE
DIAMOND
FLORITE
LAPIS LAZULI
PERIDOT
RODOCHROSITE

NERVOUS SYSTEM
MOONSTONE
OBSIDIAN/GOLDEN SHEEN
SELENITE
SODOLITE
TURQUOISE

OPENS CHAKRAS
DIAMOND—ALL
KUNZITE—FOURTH
LAPIS LAZULI—ALL
TOPAZ—SEVENTH

PANCREAS
MOONSTONE
PERIDOT
QUARTZ/CLEAR
TIGER'S EYE/YELLOW
TOURMALINE/GREEN

PITUITARY AND PINEAL GLANDS
AMETHYST
GARNET/RED
MALACHITE
MOONSTONE
SUGILITE
TOURMALINE/GREEN

SKELETAL SYSTEM
BLOODSTONE LAPIS LAZULI

SLEEP DISORDERS
MALACHITE

SPLEEN
AZURITE
BLOODSTONE
HEMATITE
MALACHITE
MOONSTONE
PERIDOT
QUARTZ/CLEAR
TIGER'S EYE/YELLOW
TOPAZ
TOURMALINE/GREEN

STOMACH/DIGESTIVE SYSTEM
TOPAZ
PYRITE
MOONSTONE

STRESS
AVENTURINE
FLORITE
HAWK'S EYE
HEMATITE
MOONSTONE
PERIDOT
TOURMALINE/GREEN

THYMUS GLAND
AQUAMARINE
QUARTZ/CLEAR

THYROID GLAND
AZURITE
CELESTITE
CHRYSOCOLLA
LAPIS LAZULI
TOURMALINE/BLUE AND GREEN

VITALITY
LAPIS LAZULI
OBSIDIAN/GOLDEN SHEEN
RUBY
SULFUR
TURQUOISE